Becoming UNSTOPPABLE WOMAN in Health & Wellness

34 HOLISTIC WAYS
TO HEAL YOUR MIND, BODY AND SOUL

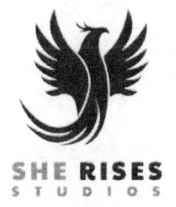

SHE RISES
STUDIOS

Hanna Olivas & Adriana Luna Carlos

Along with 32 Inspiring Women Authors

© 2022 ALL RIGHTS RESERVED.
Published by She Rises Studios Publishing www.SheRisesStudios.com.

No part of this book may be reproduced or transmitted in any form whatsoever, electronic, or mechanical, including photocopying, recording, or by any informational storage or retrieval system without the expressed written, dated and signed permission from the publisher and co-authors.

LIMITS OF LIABILITY/DISCLAIMER OF WARRANTY:

The co-authors and publisher of this book have used their best efforts in preparing this material. While every attempt has been made to verify the information provided in this book, neither the co-authors nor the publisher assumes any responsibility for any errors, omissions, or inaccuracies.

The co-authors and publisher make no representation or warranties with respect to the accuracy, applicability, or completeness of the contents of this book. They disclaim any warranties (expressed or implied), merchantability, or for any purpose. The co-authors and publisher shall in no event be held liable for any loss or other damages, including but not limited to special, incidental, consequential, or other damages.

ISBN: 979-8-9869367-5-8

Table of Contents

INTRODUCTION 7

THE JOURNEY IS PERSONAL
By Hanna Olivas 11

UNWAVERING PERSEVERANCE
By Adriana Luna Carlos 14

EVERYTHING IS ENERGI
By Priya Ali 17

FEEL IT TO HEAL IT AND DEAL WITH IT
By Angela Goday 23

DITCHING THE YO-YO LIFESTYLE
By Molly McNamee 29

SURVIVING TO THRIVING
By Katie Markel 37

THE WAR ON WEIGHT
By Keatha Landauer 43

MINDSET IS THE KEY TO WELLNESS
By Pamela Kurt 50

YOUR MIND ON BEING YOU
By Paula Echeverri 57

MONEY MADNESS & WEALTH HEALTH
By Heather Stokes Benton 63

BEING YOUR OWN ADVOCATE IN LIFE
By Colleen McCartney 70

CALL ON DOCTORS BUT PLEASE ROW AWAY FROM MEDICATIONS
By Catherine Rogers 77

OVERLOADED BUT NOT UNSTOPPABLE
By Dr. Shelby Decker 84

REBEL HEART
By Jennifer Cairns 91

THE WEALTHY MINDSET AND WELLNESS:
A HOLISTIC APPROACH TO HEALTH AND WELLNESS
By Lovely LaGuerre 98

LIVING THE DREAM THROUGH WELLNESS
By Natalie Pickett 106

I HEAR BIRDS CHIRPING
By Michele Kline 113

MOVING THE MOUNTAINS IN YOUR HEART
By Rebecca Chandler 120

BEAUTY FROM ASHES: A HEALING PATH FOR
THE MIND, BODY & SOUL
By Amanda O'Mara 127

PRIORITIZE SELF-CARE TO AVOID BURNOUT
By Natasha Ganes and Jennifer Griffith 135

HOPE'S PROMISE
By Andra Annette 141

WITH YOUR NEXT EXHALE...
By Olivia Radcliffe 149

TIME TO PULL THE REINS
By Roxana Valeton 156

EXPLORE YOUR INNER DIVA
By Krystal Vernee' 162

MIND YOUR FLOW
By Lauren Weiss 169

REIGNITE THE SPARK WITHIN

   By Rita Marrari 176

BECOME AN AGELESS GODDESS
   By Kim Rendon 182

A MENTAL HEALTH "CHECK IN" LIST FOR MOMS WITH STRUGGLING TEENS
   By Nicole Curtis 189

ATTRACT FULFILLMENT AND SUCCESS THROUGH BALANCE AND SELF-LOVE
   By Divya Chandegra 196

UNFINISHED HEALING
   By Brandi Kepley 204

LIGHT AND THE PROTECTIVE WARRIOR
   By Minh Vu 211

LIVE A FULLY CHARGED LIFE TODAY
   By Charlotte Howard Collins 222

FROM TOTAL HEALTH TRANSFORMATION TO FINANCIAL FREEDOM
   By A. Michelle Bell 228

JOIN THE MOVEMENT! #BAUW 235

INTRODUCTION

She Rises Studios was created and inspired by the mother-daughter duo Hanna Olivas and Adriana Luna Carlos. In the middle of 2020, when the world was at one of its most vulnerable times, we saw the need to embrace women globally by offering inspirational quotes, blogs, and articles. Then, in March of 2021, we launched our very own Women's Empowerment Podcast: *She Rises Studios Podcast*.

It is now one of the most sought out Women based podcasts both nationally and internationally. You can find us on your favorite podcast platforms, such as Spotify, Google Podcasts, Apple Podcasts, IHeartRadio, and much more! We didn't stop there. Establishing a safe space for women has become an even deeper need. Due to a global pandemic, women lost their businesses, employment, homes, finances, spouses, and more.

We decided to form the She Rises Studios Community Facebook Group. An environment strictly for women about women. Our focus in this group is to educate and celebrate women globally. To meet them exactly where they are on their journey.

It's a group of Ordinary Women Doing EXTRAordinary Things.

As we continued to grow our network, we saw a need to help shape the minds and influences of women struggling with insecurities, doubts, fears, etc. From this, we created a global movement known as:

Becoming An Unstoppable Woman in Health & Wellness

Every woman, at some point sooner than later, should conduct an in-depth evaluation of where they are in their health and wellness journey.

We should make resolutions before the beginning of a new year and set realistic expectations. We have to start right now where we are!

It's more important now than ever to focus on our health and wellness goals first and foremost. It should be one of our top priorities in our lives. Without our health, what good is our wealth?

Society has created many stigmas about how women should look, feel, and function.

These stigmas have caused women to become stressed, anxious, overwhelmed, overweight, and suffer from mental and physical disorders.

We want to change those stigmas, kill the information overload button, and provide truth to this arena. That is why women worldwide have shared their journeys to optimal health and overall well-being in this book.

These women have made it their life's passion and purpose to elevate and educate other women to do the same. Let's focus on being the best healthy version of ourselves. You can achieve your goals with hope, dedication, perseverance, and consistency.

Becoming An Unstoppable Woman in Health and Wellness is the perfect guide to get you started. You get a fantastic book with 30-plus strategies and a community of women who want you to succeed and have optimal health.

This is more than a book. It's a movement!
Join the #BAUW team today.

Start living an abundant and powerful life!

She Rises Studios offers:

- She Rises Studios Publishing
- She Rises Studios Public Relations
- She Rises Studios Podcast
- She Rises Studios Magazine

- Becoming An Unstoppable Woman TV Show
- She Rises Studios Community
- She Rises Studios Academy

We won't stop encouraging women to be Unstoppable. This is just the beginning of our global movement.

She Rises, She Leads, She Lives...

With Love,
HANNA OLIVAS
ADRIANA LUNA CARLOS
SHE RISES STUDIOS
www.sherisesstudios.com

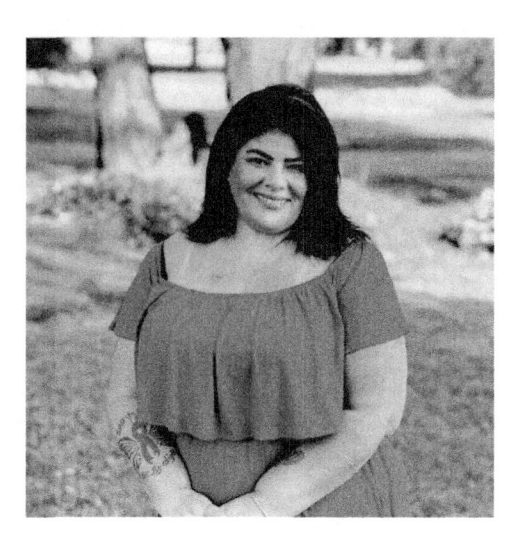

Hanna Olivas

Founder & CEO of She Rises Studios
Podcast & TV Host | Best Selling Author | Influential Speaker | Blood Cancer Advocate | #BAUW Movement Creator

https://www.linkedin.com/company/she-rises-studios/
https://www.instagram.com/sherisesstudios/
https://www.facebook.com/sherisesstudios
www.SheRisesStudios.com

Author, Speaker, and Founder. Hanna was born and raised in Las Vegas, Nevada, and has paved her way to becoming one of the most influential women of 2023. Hanna is the co-founder of She Rises Studios and the founder of the Brave & Beautiful Blood Cancer Foundation. Her journey started in 2017 when she was first diagnosed with Multiple Myeloma, an incurable blood cancer. Now more than ever, her focus is to empower other women to become leaders because The Future is Female. She is currently traveling and speaking publicly to women to educate them on entrepreneurship, leadership, and owning the female power within.

THE JOURNEY IS PERSONAL

By Hanna Olivas

To the women who read this book, we hope you will be inspired and empowered to choose your health and wellness as your first priority. It is such a vital choice and a pivotal moment in your life. We, as women, are being diagnosed with chronic disease, pain, anxiety, depression, cancer, obesity, and other health problems.

The only way to stop those is to take control of our mental and physical health. This book isn't magic. It's a guide to assist you in making positive changes that are so desperately needed. We've seen a shift in women not wanting to do self-care or even have healthy sleeping habits.

We often become robots in a routine of always being on the go. Stopping at the nearest fast food joint because we tell ourselves we don't have time to cook. We continue to choose less sleep to make money or continuously operate in fight or flight mode. Our question is, when is it enough? What changes can you make immediately to avoid stress, burnout, or even a dam heart attack? Will you leave that stressful situation or will you seek help? That's the other issue; women don't like to ask for help.

A lot of us suffer in silence and mental or physical anguish. It's time to focus on living a happy and healthy life. Please don't wait until it's too late. Your time is now!

Inside this book are so many different stories of women who have overcome some of life's biggest health and mental health problems. They have chosen to share their journey with you.

Often we need that extra push, that accountability partner; however, you are the only one who can choose to unleash your true optimal health and wellness. We encourage you as you read each chapter to focus and understand the power of a woman on a mission for change.

Know that these women are a true testimony that it can be done. Start choosing yourself and start your journey of Becoming An Unstoppable Woman In Health and Wellness.

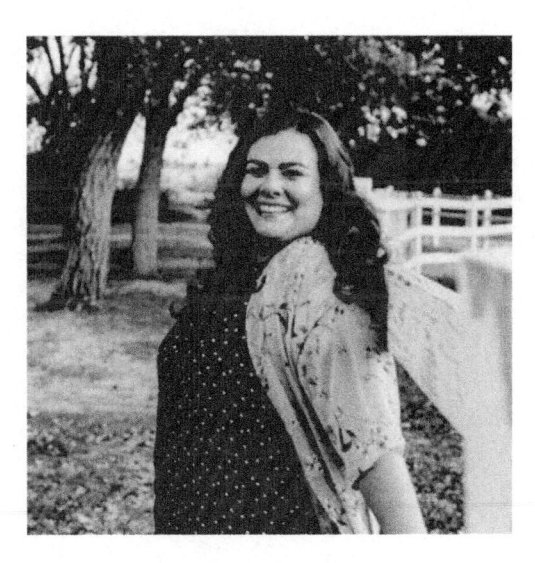

Adriana Luna Carlos

Founder & CEO of She Rises Studios
Podcast Host | Best Selling Author | #BAUW Movement Creator

https://www.linkedin.com/company/she-rises-studios/
https://www.instagram.com/sherisesstudios/
https://www.facebook.com/sherisesstudios
www.SheRisesStudios.com

Adriana Luna Carlos is a much sought-after expert in Web and Graphic design as well as a new Podcast Host Personnel for She Rises Studios. For over 10 years she has embraced her passion in the digital arts field along with helping women worldwide overcome their insecure idiosyncrasies. Today, when she's not spending time with her family and friends, you'll often find her helping woman focus on rising up and becoming unafraid of success. To learn more about Adriana Luna Carlos and how she can help you overcome obstacles in your business, mindset, or insecurities, visit www.SheRisesStudios.com

UNWAVERING PERSEVERANCE

By Adriana Luna Carlos

Unwavering perseverance is what makes a woman unstoppable in nurturing her well-being. To do so, you have to take care of yourself physically and also leap into a deeper sense of understanding of who you are.

Constantly, you will face uncertainties and hurdles as you go about your daily life. Instead of taking them negatively, embrace them as an opportunity to develop yourself.

Just like the women who shared their stories in this book, thrive to move forward. They were able to rise over unfavorable occasions because they believed in themselves.

If you put your mind in everything you do, you'd be able overcome even the most extreme impact of feeling down, stressed, fatigued, anxious, and other tough circumstances.

There is an adage that says "Experience is the best teacher." With regards, this book contains first-hand experiences of triumphant women that will inspire you to never give up and pursue a healthy life.

Take the first step by empowering yourself through women's stories. After all, only by motivating yourself would you be able to also steer other women toward success.

When you change the way you see things, you become strong. The more you seek the good in everything, the more likely you will be able to live your life to the fullest.

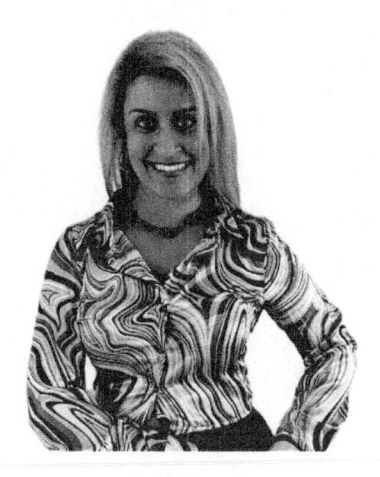

Priya Ali

Founder & CEO of Energi Living 365 Wellness Group

www.linkedin.com/in/priya-ali-3237487
https://www.instagram.com/startliving365
https://www.facebook.com/priya.ali
www.living365wellness.love
www.energi.love

Priya Ali is a dedicated entrepreneur and mother of four babies. She has led a successful personal and executive coaching practice, Energi Living 365, since 2007.

After dropping out of high school at the age of 17, she quickly developed her entrepreneurial skills and never looked back. Energi Living 365, is dedicated to enabling dramatic personal and professional growth amongst its clients. Through highly personalized coaching and guidance, Energi Living 365 empowers clients to establish positive, productive thought processes and behaviors.

Priya also possesses unique intuitive abilities as a third generation intuitive, healer, and medium that she applies in each of her service offerings. This intuitive capacity allows her to quickly extract valuable insights from individuals and social groups, providing clients with guidance that is both objective and keenly insightful.

Priya Ali has cultivated her natural talent through a wide range of professional certifications and accreditation to maximize her capacity to support the personal, professional, spiritual and physical goals of her clients.

EVERYTHING IS ENERGI

By Priya Ali

From the time I was five I found that I could see into people's beings. I would see different colors of lights in and around them. If my mom or dad had pain, I would look inside their bodies and would see what appeared to be black matter, and it would be in the location of their pain. It wasn't until my 20s that I gained clear awareness of my gifts as an empath, intuitive, and healer. I began using my gifts to start a career as a reader and healer in my 30s. I was able to read energies, remove negative energies, cleanse energies, and balance energies. As a result, I had clients who were pleased with their results and the noticeable improvements or positive changes they were experiencing. They would be on their merry way, but then they would come back, three, six, or twelve months later with the same types of issues, ailments, or challenges. It was both perplexing and irritating to me that the results did not have more permanence.

I sought guidance and clarity through meditation and came to the awareness that while we can work on our non-physical selves, we have to look at our physical selves as well. All disharmony and disease begin in the energetic fields of the etheric body. If we don't address the day-to-day life issues that we experience, the energy of those issues goes unprocessed and eventually becomes toxic. If these toxic energies remain in the etheric body for a long time, they penetrate the physical layers of the body, leading to disease. The signs of disharmony can be seen through the negative emotions we experience, such as fear, anger, heartache, insecurity, and resentment, to name a few. Once this became apparent to me, I partnered with a functional medicine doctor. I would tell him the areas of the body I would see disharmony in, I would do the energetic healing and he would work with the clients on the physical healing. Once again, with the two of us working together, we had clients who were pleased with their results and the noticeable improvements or positive changes they were experiencing, and once again they would come back three, six, or twelve months later with the same types of issues, ailments, or challenges. There was a change in how deeply they were affected, it wasn't as bad as before, but the changes were still not sustainable.

I returned to meditation to gain more guidance and clarity, this time coming to a new awareness. The guidance that came through to me is something I already knew: we are a body, mind, and spirit. As such, we need congruence with these three elements. If we make a change to one element, we have to bring the other two elements up to speed. Otherwise, the elements that haven't changed will pull the one or two elements that have changed back down. Since I had mastered working with spirit and body, the next logical step was to work on the mind. At this time, I began to study mindset, neuroscience, neuro-linguistic programming, and the brain, and connected to the fact that our body, mind, and spirit each have their own energy and each one is operating from those energies.

This led me to create a very customized approach to working with my clients. Most traditional western medicine remedies are not customized to any one person, but rather to the masses. It's easy to see that our physiology can impact the effectiveness of a western medicine remedy.

This means that a pill may affect us differently if, for example, we are sleep deprived and dehydrated, then it would be if we were well-rested and fully hydrated. Oftentimes we don't connect that same theory to our mind and spirit, but they are equally impacted if not sometimes more. Our physiology can impact our minds and spirits too. Each element of your being has a vibration that impacts your thoughts and feelings concerning each topic and area in your life experience. By having an awareness and understanding of the vibrations each element of your being is emitting, you allow yourself the opportunity to adjust, make changes, and bring your mind, body, and spirit into alignment.

Once I began to implement this new strategy, we saw the all too familiar clients who were pleased with their results and the noticeable improvements or positive changes they were experiencing. The difference was the results seemed to be permanent for the most part. On the way to obtaining these results, one of the things I began to notice was how different thoughts created different energies within a person, some being negative and some being positive. As I began to dig deeper, I could see how some thoughts were actually leading the clients toward illness. Have you ever said, or heard someone else say, "Just the thought of it makes me sick?" At the time, you or that person may not have meant it literally, but it can happen. Repeatedly thinking negative thoughts can create negativity not only in your mind but in your body and spirit as well. Recently, we have been heavily encouraged to "Just think positive thoughts!" The challenge with this: is if you don't actually believe it, if you don't actually feel the positivity in your spirit and your body, your positive energy and thoughts will be overshadowed by this disbelief and lack of feeling

As clients began healing and were able to create permanent change, we started focusing on prevention. Most people will go to the gym, start losing weight, and then stop going to the gym. Continuing the process that leads you to heal is imperative to prevent a new occurrence. This applies to ailments of all elements of your being, your mind, your body, and your spirit. Most people get that when it comes to their bodies, but many don't make the association to their minds and spirit. Notice that I used the term "new occurrence" rather than recurrence or relapse. That is because, once we have healed an ailment or affliction, it will not repeat unless we create it again. Liken it to pregnancy: once a woman goes through the phases of pregnancy and postpartum, she will not relapse into pregnancy. She has to create the condition of pregnancy again by repeating the steps she took the first time.

Everything is energy. If you were to examine the device or paper you are reading this chapter on under a microscope, you would see the atoms, molecules, and fibers that they are composed of to make up the solid matter. Similarly, our beings are composed of cells and our bodies run on chemical energy. The way that we think, speak, act, receive our information, and respond in our interactions all have an energy, and that energy plays a vital part in our well-being, or lack thereof. The energy we engage in when performing activities can affect the outcomes of those activities. Take eating a meal for example. For a few days, eat your dinner with a violent action or horror movie playing on TV, then for a few days, eat your dinner with classical or soft music playing in the background and observe the differences in your digestion. Consuming your food while experiencing stress can actually put stressed energy into your food, and as you digest, process, and eliminate that food, that stressful energy interacts with your body as it digests.

By assisting my clients with awareness of the energies of their mind, body, and spirit and customizing a process for healing and balance, together we have seen noticeable changes such as facial paralysis reversed, loss of eyesight restored, tumors shrink, and recovery from eating disorders, substance abuse, addictions, anxiety, and depression to name just a few. There is no "one size fits all" remedy for anything or anyone, which is why it is important for you to educate yourself about your own mind, body, and spirit. When you access your innate, intuitive ability to be tuned in and tapped into you, you can become your own healer. You will also be able to advocate for your well-being when necessary. How many times have you personally experienced, or heard of someone else experiencing, a physician or health practitioner say there is nothing wrong, when in fact there was? When we know ourselves, we know when something is off, or when something has changed. If we pay attention to the frequent headaches, pains in our bodies, and changes in our physical abilities, mental disposition, or energies rather than ignoring them, or silencing those warning symptoms by medicating them, we give ourselves the chance to avoid further decline in our well-being. Living your life with an understanding that everything is energy will allow you to live from a place of heightened awareness of the things, people, and experiences that will support you in living a life of well-being.

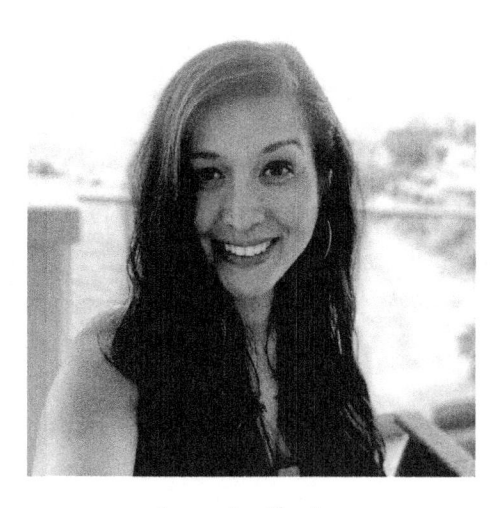

Angela Goday

Founder of Serenity and Salud

https://www.instagram.com/serenityandsalud/
https://serenityandsaludhangout.com/

Angela is the founder of Serenity and Salud, a Spiritual Yoga Coach and Transformative Travel Designer. Serenity and Salud shows women how to reclaim their wellness, create their own calm, and live their life in alignment with love. As a Multiple Myeloma survivor, Angela knows first hand the importance of caring for your mind, body and soul. She incorporates Yoga, spirituality, and travel to help women transcend from the aftermath of a cancer diagnosis and reset their nervous system. Her personal experience of reconnecting with her body, and soul through travel, inspired her to show other women how to do the same. Angela designs transformative travel trips for women who are on a soul searching journey. Her signature program Epic Escapes is a tailored travel approach for those with unique wellness needs. Her mission is to help women venture out and within.

FEEL IT TO HEAL IT AND DEAL WITH IT

By Angela Goday

I became attracted to Yoga because I have always been physically flexible. When I attended my first Yoga teacher training I discovered the immense amount of off the mat and spiritual benefits Yoga has to offer. Flaunting the body's flexibility and assuming pretzel-like postures was the easy part. I didn't know that Yoga would show me how to have mental flexibility and stay grounded when life circumstances were beyond my control. My Yoga practice became a lifeline for me when I had surgeries that limited my physical mobility. Yoga showed me how to self-regulate and cope with my chronic cancer. Throughout the years, my yoga practice has evolved and become the greatest catalyst for my personal transformation. I learned to venture within to transcend my physical limitations. Yoga is the key I use to access my inner calm. I use what I have learned on the Yoga mat to help me spiritually feel, heal, and deal with life off the mat. I am excited to share with you how Yoga goes beyond physical, along with tools you can use to feel, heal and deal with life off the mat.

Feel It: Alignment

Yoga teaches us the importance of alignment. Having properly aligned physical posture is important for protecting the integrity of the spine and preventing injury. Alignment is internal and external and what we look like and feel like. In life, when we are not aligned with who we are, we jeopardize our integrity and block our energy flow. Have you ever noticed those areas of your life that seem effortless? That is what it looks and feels like when you are in alignment both in a Yoga pose and in life. When we are out of alignment with who we are, it is hard to listen to our intuition and trust our own decisions. In today's world, it is so easy to lose connection to our intuition. We are constantly bombarded with social media images and energies that we pick up from other people, so we start to become confused and out of alignment with who we truly are. We are all divinely and uniquely made, which is why we all look different even though we are doing the same yoga pose. When we compare our journey to someone else's we become distracted from remembering who we truly are. Yoga helps you make a conscious connection that you can feel between your body and your internal world. You can experience alignment on and off the mat.

Feel It: Off the Mat Spiritual Tool

Take a moment to recall a positive experience where you were in a complete energetic flow. The experience can be anything, like a relationship or a project you were working on. What bodily sensations did you feel? Did you feel a sense of expansion and aliveness? Do the sensations have a color? On a piece of paper, draw a gingerbread man shaped body and color inside where you felt the sensations. Next, label the names of the sensations. Now you have a reference for future reflection. For comparison, you can also do this for a negative experience. Becoming aware of the sensations you feel in your body is essential for discerning when something is right for you and in alignment with who you truly are.

Heal It: Learning to Let Go

Breathwork is a fundamental part of Yoga. Deep body stretches accompanied by deep breathing help release and break up stagnant tissue in the body. Breathwork practices have taught me how to physically and spiritually release and let go. Before I do anything that requires me to dig deep and find courage, I spend a few minutes focusing on my breath. It's my superpower for calming and soothing my anxious nervous system. So much stress, anxiety, and even physical tension can be relieved with proper diaphragmatic breathing. Sometimes, reminding myself to breathe is the only healing tool I have when something becomes difficult. There are so many different forms of breathwork you can explore. The best part about breathwork is that you can practice it anywhere; you don't need to be in a fancy yoga studio or use any props. Becoming aware of your breath is the first step. Begin by placing one hand on your belly and one hand on your chest. You should feel your belly expanding and contracting as you breathe. If not, then you are most likely breathing in a shallow manner from your chest. If you have ever had a panic attack, then you know that feeling of gasping for air and breathing from your chest instead of your belly. Now that you are aware of your breath and how it's a powerful self-healing tool, let's look at how we can use it off the mat.

Heal It: Off the Mat Spiritual Tool

Five finger breath practice: Before you begin, set an intention of what you want to release and let go of. For this practice, you can choose to keep your eyes open or closed. Use one hand to trace the fingers on your opposite hand. As you trace each finger upwards, inhale through your nose, then trace each finger downwards and exhale through your nose. As you inhale, imagine yourself healing and absorbing all of the qualities of your highest self. When you exhale, visualize yourself letting go of whatever is holding you back. You can visualize letting go of pain, a relationship, or a situation that you can't control. Just taking one or two minutes to do this can have a profound effect on the rest of your day.

Finding Ways To: Deal With It

One of my favorite quotes comes from a famous Yogi and teacher B.K.S. Iyengar. He says that "Yoga teaches us to cure what need not be endured and endure what cannot be cured."

This quote reminds me that different circumstances call for different measures. I learned that healing is not quantifiable, and there are no boxes to check off. You have to explore different modalities to discover what works best for you. Some of the modalities I have explored include Art Therapy, Writing Therapy, EFT Tapping, Affirmative Prayer, Meditation, Mindfulness, Sensory Stimulation, Spiritual Travel, and, of course, Yoga. Yoga works for me because I tend to spend way too much time burning up energy in my head. I crave grounding and re-centering exercises to help me reconnect and move out of my head and into my body. Living with chronic cancer encourages me to think outside of the box and find tools I can use that aren't physical. I need tools for the days when I just don't have any physical strength.

One of the tools that I use is what I call the Five Senses Self-Soothing Survival Kit. It's a technique from Dialectical Behavior Therapy and is used for people who have emotion dysregulation disorder. When I discovered this, I knew I needed it because after my cancer diagnosis I experienced a flood of uncontrollable and unpredictable emotions and I needed to find a way to heal. As you know, our five senses include touch, taste, sight, smell, and hearing. Focusing on your five senses shifts the focus from your thoughts to your bodily sensations. I keep my survival kit in a beautiful basket in my closet filled with things like coloring books, fuzzy socks, tea bags, note cards with healthy reminders, essential oils, gum, mints, spiritual books, and kinesthetic sand. When I'm anxious I love to pick up kinesthetic sand and squish it between my hands. It helps me slow my thoughts down and brings me a sense of calm. Touching the sand grounds me, places me in the present moment, and affirms my nervous system that I am safe. Let's look at how you can create your own Self Soothing Survival Kit to help you create inner calm, and deal with life off the yoga mat.

Deal With It: Off the Mat Spiritual Tool

Create your own Five Senses Self-Soothing Survival Kit. Find a pretty basket you can keep your things in, or use wrapping paper to wrap up an old box you have lying around the house. For the items in your basket, gather one thing for each of your five senses: smell, taste, touch, sight, and hearing. Some examples are essential oil, kinesthetic sand, indulgent chocolate, a memorable picture or postcard, and a playlist that elicits the emotion you want to feel like happy, fun, or maybe even sad.

I believe that health and wellness are about exploring different paths and keeping them in a mental toolbox or a physical box that you can pull out when you need it. My business name is Serenity and Salud, and it was chosen with great intention. In Spanish, salud means health. I help women find serenity and salud to reclaim their wellness with Yoga, spiritual practices, and transformative travel experiences. When you are ready to explore any of these modalities please visit serenityandsaludhangout.com to get in contact with me and view my current offerings.

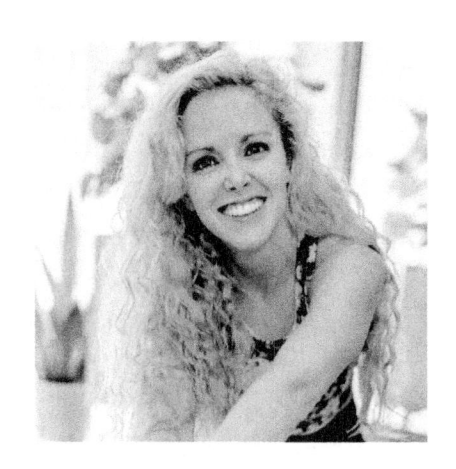

Molly McNamee

Founder of MFit Workouts

https://www.instagram.com/mfit.workouts/
https://www.facebook.com/itsmollyrae
https://www.linkedin.com/in/molly-mcnamee-81718699/
https://mollymcnamee.com/

Molly is an online health and fitness coach. She created MFit in 2013 and has expanded it over the years to become an online gym experience where people get workouts and health coaching from her website. MFit has allowed Molly to work with clients from all over the world.

Movement has always been a part of Molly's life. She did competitive dance and gymnastics through her child and teen years and grew up in a sports-loving family, playing a myriad of sports with her brothers.

She took this passion for movement and became a certified personal trainer in 2013. Since then she has gotten further certifications in sports nutrition, corrective exercise, women's health, and more.

Her goal as a trainer is to help people break out of the yo-yo cycle that many find themselves stuck in. She helps her clients create sustainable fitness routines that leave them feeling confident and strong!

DITCHING THE YO-YO LIFESTYLE

By Molly McNamee

Let's Start From the Beginning

I have been "exercising" since I was a little girl. I got involved in gymnastics and dance at the young age of five, which meant I was regularly conditioning my body for 3+ hours every day all through primary and secondary school.

This is acceptable as a kid. Kids can run around all day and feel *more* energized for it. But we don't stay kids forever. Both our minds and our bodies change as we get older. And that change hit me hard.

As I moved into my teen years, I became very aware of my changing body. I gained some curves and lost some confidence. Puberty created a lot of body image issues for me, as it does for many girls. Ultimately, I became obsessed with what I ate so that I could control how my body looked. I'll be honest, I didn't eat very much. And I was still exercising a whole lot. So, my weight dropped down to 80 pounds.

Yikes.

It's safe to say that I took that need to control my body too far, but as a teen, I was able to bounce back quickly. I recognized that I had an issue. I started eating more and gained the weight I needed back.

However, we don't stay teenagers forever, and the next time I gained and lost weight wasn't quite as easy.

I moved to Los Angeles when I was 19 years old. After the move, I struggled to balance my new life with health and fitness. As a result, I gained 40 pounds. I knew I didn't want to get back into my old disordered eating habits, so I started going to the gym instead.

You're thinking: good for you! But, no, we aren't there yet. Stay with me!

I lost those 40 pounds and then continued to gain and lose 10-20 pounds every few months for the next seven years. My energy, confidence, and motivation went up and down every few months too.

About a year after I started working out at the gym, I got my personal training certification, and suddenly fitness was a bigger part of my life than it had ever been before. It was not only my job but my wellness and my personal time too.

If I could go back and tell younger Molly something, it would be "practice what you preach." Because I definitely didn't do that.

I always told my clients that they needed a sustainable workout routine. One that they could do without falling off or feeling burnt out. But, guess what I was doing…?

I would jump from one extreme to the next. I had no concept of balance.

I worked out hard for several hours a day, every single day. I would do cardio and strength and Yoga. I would watch what I ate — eating plenty of vegetables and protein. I loved the way I looked and felt. I was strong and lean.

Well, every other month that is.

I'm not exaggerating when I say that I would go from feeling energized in that routine one day to feeling completely drained and bloated the next day.

And that feeling would last several weeks. In those weeks when I felt tired and unmotivated, I would gain weight. Oftentimes a lot of weight.

This may sound crazy, but I didn't even realize this was a problem. I always eventually got my energy back. I was able to get back to my crazy routine and lose whatever weight I had gained during my weeks of retrograde. Sure, I constantly felt like I was starting over. But I helped new clients start over every day. It didn't seem like a big deal. So, I let this pattern go on for seven years. Feeling heavy, weak, worn out, and lazy every couple of months.

And then I stopped going to the gym. Not by choice, but by injury.

I hit my head and got a concussion and was no longer physically able to continue this all-or-nothing lifestyle I had going on. I wish it didn't take a concussion to break me out of it, but it did.

I was no longer able to do the types of nor the quantity of workouts I was doing. So, I started doing low-impact cardio and strength workouts at home. I went from working out 3+ hours a day, as I'd been doing since I was a kid, to 40-minutes a day max.

And suddenly, I felt really good. Better than I ever felt before. I was able to maintain my results indefinitely. That tired, burnt-out, and bloated feeling never came back. Three years later, this is still true. I am as strong as I was, as lean as I was, and as confident as I was during those "good" periods of going to the gym with none of the fallout.

Now, you may or may not see yourself in parts of my story. However, a lot of adults find themselves in this yo-yo cycle that I was stuck in for seven years. The cycle of gaining and losing the same 15 pounds over and over again, of constantly feeling tired and unmotivated to exercise and having to always "start over" when it comes to their fitness — feeling a lack of control over their bodies.

I made it out of this yo-yo lifestyle. And I learned a lot in the process. So, now I've made it my mission to help others break out of the yo-yo pattern too.

Ending the Yo-yo Cycle

I don't want you to have to experience a debilitating concussion to break out of your yo-yo lifestyle. So, I've created a 3-step system to end the cycle healthily.

Step 1: Start Moving

To snap out of the all-or-nothing mentality, you need to make movement a normal part of your day. I want you to stop associating movement with hour-long workouts at 5AM. Movement is so much more than that.

When you start moving your body more, you feel less pressured to do aggressive workout programs. You no longer need to out-exercise a sedentary life.

Making your life more active is going to improve your energy too. You'll feel more awake, productive, and motivated. Which will help you be more alert at work, positive for your family, and happier overall.

The first thing I have all of my clients do is find ways to sneak movement into their day-to-day that doesn't feel disruptive. Because, again, we want movement to feel normal, not like something that should be viewed as a chore or something extreme.

Here are a few of my favorite ways to be more active.

I like to call this first strategy the Alert Method. Anytime you get an alert on your phone, fix your posture. This will take a second of your time, but if you turn all alerts on and your phone goes off 50 times during the day, you're suddenly moving a lot more. Engaging your core and postural muscles a lot more and actively thinking about your body throughout the day. Which is exactly what we want.

Speaking of the phone, walk around while you chat on your cell.

Admittedly, if you work in an office, this may not be easy. But, could you squeeze your abs while you chat instead?

Finally, start multitasking. March in place as you microwave your food. Do calf raises as you brush your teeth. Think about those moments in your day when you're doing something that takes very little effort and ask yourself how you can be active while you do those things.

Step 2: Ease Into a Routine

The biggest mistake I see people make on their fitness journey is doing too much too soon. You wouldn't go from barely walking to running a marathon in a week, so why would you go from not exercising at all to going to the gym every single day?

You need to ease into it. You should start by doing three structured workouts a week, where the workouts are only 10-15 minutes long. Then, build off of that routine. As your body gets used to it, make the workouts a little longer. Then add a fourth workout into the mix.

Your current body cannot do the types of workouts that you want your "goal body" to be able to do. So, work with what you got. Start small and then build. Do not overwhelm your current body. Because if you do too much too soon, you are going to fall off. And when you fall off, the yo-yo cycle begins again.

Step 3: Don't Start Something You Can't do Forever

If there is an end date to your fitness program or diet, then there is also an end date to your results. If you want to stop yo-yoing, you need to stop thinking about health and fitness as a short-term thing.

You should never go into a new routine thinking, "I could do this for a couple months." You need to be willing to follow that routine forever, or at least for the foreseeable future. Remember what I said in step two: if there is a falloff point, the yo-yo cycle begins again.

If you think you can do the routine forever but find yourself falling off every couple of months as I did, then you're not doing the right program.

Now, this isn't to say you can't go on vacation and ditch your routine for a week. However, if you go on vacation it should be incredibly easy for you to get back into your routine because it is that rooted in your life.

This process isn't easy by any means. We are talking about transforming your life and the way your brain thinks about wellness, but if you ease into it, take away the intimidation factor of fitness, and focus on building a routine you can have for life, you'll get there.

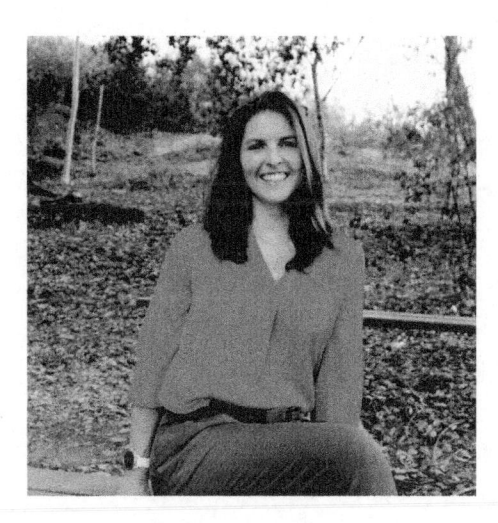

Katie Markel

CEO/Founder of She Eats

https://www.facebook.com/groups/435228411705256
https://www.instagram.com/kd.nbalance/
https://www.sheeatslifestyle.com/

Podcast: She Eats Lifestyle
https://open.spotify.com/show/4VbdiTYFFcASyx8g2fAyfO

I am a Kinesiologist, Nutrition Coach, Hormone Specialist, Holistic Health Practitioner, Corrective Exercise Specialist, Personal Trainer, Massage Therapist, and Marine Veteran.

I am the CEO of She Eats, a women's holistic health company.

The goal of She Eats is to support women in living their healthiest and happiest lives through cycle synced nutrition and fitness. She Eats is a community of amazing women that meet online. We work as a group or in one-on-one coaching sessions.

She Eats can be found on Facebook, Instagram, Spotify and Apple Music, under the She Eats Community.

She Eats is on a mission to inform and empower women to have maximized health by understanding how their unique hormone levels are related to metabolism and nutrition. She Eats teaches women to fuel their bodies and get results in half the time while eating more, doing less, and never missing out on a moment of life.

SURVIVING TO THRIVING

By Katie Markel

I haven't met a woman who hasn't tried at least one diet.

She's tried cutting out carbs, only eating 1200 calories, or doing a cardio class every day. She's taken on challenges with her husband only for him to continue seeing progress while she plateaued, or worse… went backward. Confused and fed up with missing out on life she quit and decided just to eat healthily. Except now, even at 1600 calories, she is still gaining weight.

She was told she isn't trying hard enough. She's not counting her calories right.

Except no one told her the truth. There is a better way for women. That women's hormones are the missing piece that has been ignored for years to make weight loss and management easy for women!

Not only weight management, but the ability to say goodbye to PMS forever! Goodbye to low energy, anxiety, and brain fog. Hello to a lifestyle that isn't a "diet," that doesn't require her to give up foods she loves. That doesn't require her to spend torturous hours on the treadmill, using up her precious energy exchanging calories burned for calories earned. Instead, she found a way that empowers and educates her on how to work with her unique body and menstrual cycle.

What She found wasn't a diet. She found a lifestyle. She found She Eats.

If this isn't you, if you don't want a sustainable way to manage weight, that is easy, enjoyable, and works with your body, then I totally understand and you can just skip this chapter.

If this is you, then I am excited to share the She Eats method.

So excited that I will give you the entire framework for this program for free!

Surviving:

Since the 80s women have been told to eat less and move more—that thigh gaps and collar bones were the epitome of health. Our menstrual cycle was a taboo event that just occurs every month. Combine these and it's no wonder women everywhere have been struggling with body image and dysfunctional relationships with food.

It wasn't until the last decade that researchers realized there was a massive disparity in the research on women. When researchers finally conducted studies on how women's hormones affect the way we process and utilize nutrients the results were game-changing!

As our hormones change throughout each month, so does our body's preference for carbs or fats for energy. The amount of protein we need also fluctuates, as well as specific nutrients we need to ward off bloating, fatigue, acne, cramps, and all other 166 symptoms of PMS you have been told are a fact of life during each month.

What this meant for women was a whole new script on "dieting."

That woman should NOT BE FOLLOWING ONE "DIET" all the time.

Instead, women should learn to work with their hormones.

One thing I have learned on this journey is that a lot of women have never been taught about the importance of their hormones. That there is more than just bleed and no bleed times, that there are key fluctuations throughout the month.

You may know, you have four phases to your menstrual cycle; menstrual, follicular, ovulation, and luteal. The two main sex hormones are estrogen and progesterone. Estrogen runs the show in your follicular phase, peaking right before ovulation and rising again in the middle of your luteal phase. Progesterone runs the show in your luteal phase, peaking mid-luteal phase.

Here is a really cool part of the story: With these predictable fluctuations in hormones, we get to try all the diets! We actually have more metabolic flexibility than men and don't need to corner ourselves into one way of eating. In fact, that is the worst thing we can do!

Even better, Estrogen loves carbs! It increases our insulin sensitivity. Estrogen plays a role in making us better at utilizing carbs. Yes, ladies! I want you to eat carbs! No more feeling like bread is the enemy, and no more getting the salad instead. No more feeling like you can't enjoy the foods you love and feel good too.

What we have to do is learn to time eating with our hormones!

When we learn to time our nutrition and fitness with our unique hormone cycles we take control. Fat loss and weight management become easy and we make progress twice as fast! But this isn't just about weight loss or physical performance. When you learn to tailor your nutrition and fitness to your cycle and you give your body what it needs, PMS disappears. The bloating, cramping, fatigue, acne, and mood swings—all gone. When you learn to work with your cycle perimenopause and menopause won't be so bad.

Thriving:

I want to share with you how I and other women have gone from *surviving* on low-calorie, low-carb, restrictive diets and doing hours of cardio to *thriving* and eating double the calories and carbs while spending half the time in the gym.

All with hormone, cycle syncing.

Let's break down the basics. Then, if you want to learn how to turn health into a lifestyle that works with your body instead of white-knuckling your way against it, you can download my free gift at the end of this chapter and start applying this for yourself.

Step 1: Tracking your cycle!

I have found that most women don't know where they are in their cycle, when the next one is coming, or why that even matters. Knowing where you are in your cycle will not only help you cycle sync your nutrition and fitness to optimize your health and ditch PMS, but it also acts as a massive health indicator of hormone balance throughout your body. I know another amazing author is talking about how to optimize your life and work schedule around your cycle as well. So make sure to check her chapter out. Some great apps to help you track and learn to track your cycle are FEMM, Clue, MyFlo, and Flo. Understanding your hormones is the key to unlocking endless possibilities in your health, wellness, and life.

Step 2: Cycle Syncing

You have probably heard of carb cycling, but *carb timing* is more important. It is timed with your unique cycle. Like I mentioned earlier, estrogen and carbs are besties. When estrogen is high in the mid–late follicular and mid–luteal phases your carbs should be high. Your body is a carb-burning machine! Give it what it wants! Feed your body and feed your soul!

When estrogen is low, we need to be a little smarter with our carb choices. This is especially critical in the late luteal phase. Keeping sugar and highly processed carbs to a minimum during this week will keep cramps, acne, bloating, and mood swings at bay. When estrogen is low, our body is not as good at utilizing carbs so the sugar remains in our bloodstream longer. This can lead to the aforementioned symptoms as well as weight gain if the excess sugar gets stored as fat, so knowing when the right time to eat carbs is powerful.

But when estrogen isn't the star, progesterone is running the show in the luteal phase and you are a fat-burning machine! Progesterone is amazing at helping you free up stored fat and burn it for energy! This is an amazing time to work in some easy cardio workouts and throw in some low-carb days to tap into your fat-burning potential. During this time, protein is critical! Just like with carbs the week before your period, fat and protein selection during this time is important. Aim for low saturated fats a week to a week and a half before your next period to ward off PMS.

Step 3: Lifestyle

The She Eats Method isn't a diet. It's a lifestyle. By adopting the She Eats Lifestyle you will master eating and training with your cycle. You will love how you feel in your skin. You feel more present, less anxious, and less fearful of what others think about your body. You never have to miss out on an experience or moment again. You are confident, proud, feeling sexy, and confident in your skin and ability to maintain what you have learned. You are officially thriving!

She Eats is on a mission to change the way women view dieting. Ending toxic dieting culture and replacing it with a culture that empowers and fuels women to be their healthiest and happiest selves.

The She Eats Community is on a mission to change the lives of millions of women. Thank you for taking the time to read my chapter. If you found value in it please share it with another woman who you think could use this too. Every woman deserves to feel her best!

If you want to implement this easy and transformative lifestyle, go to www.katiesfreegift.com to download the entire framework for free!

Join the free community at www.facebook.com/sheeats
Instagram: she.eats.lifestyle
Podcast: She Eats Lifestlye

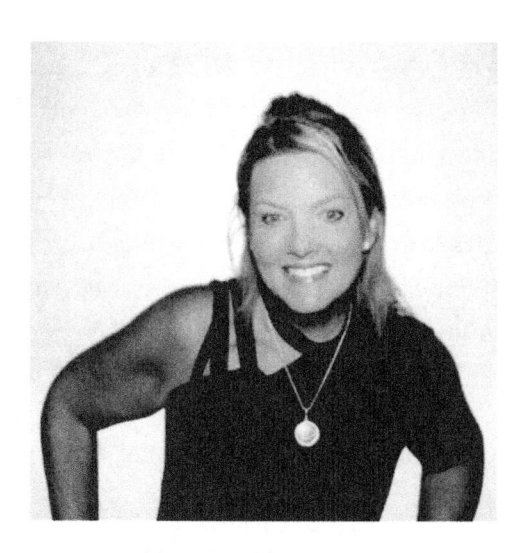

Keatha Landauer

PodcastHost: The War on Weight
Speaker, Trainer, Wellness Instructor and Coach

https://www.facebook.com/keatha.Leann.Landauer
https://www.instagram.com/keatha_landauer/
https://coachkeatha.com/
https://thewaronweight.com

Author, Speaker, Podcast Host, Wife, Mom, Coach, coffee drinking, lipstick loving Jesus Freak. After almost 30 years of battling her weight and eating dysfunction she's won the war on her weight. She now has a passion to help other women do the same. On her podcast, The War On Weight, she gives her listeners many resources for total transformation in their health, happiness, and confidence. When working with Keatha as a one-to-one client, you'll find support, accountability, and your biggest cheerleader. Keatha is a coach that has battled her own weight and can relate to your pain and frustration over the bathroom scale. She has simple solutions for you that win your own war on weight.

THE WAR ON WEIGHT

By Keatha Landauer

If you've battled your weight at all, you know it feels like an all-out WAR. I know it did for me, and it started from a very early age. My battle started with thoughts of "What's wrong with you?", "Why do people leave?", "Why don't people like you?", and "You don't fit in." Those negative thoughts on repeat, in addition to early years of dieting and not knowing how to process life events and feelings of being unworthy, led me to secret eating and binge eating. Once you get yourself in the diet, binge, overexercise, overeat, and then the new diet of the week cycle, it begins to feel overwhelming and eventually you become a prisoner in your own body. Living for more than 30 years in this brutal cycle led to many poor choices, beating myself up in my head over and over and feeling like a failure no matter what I did. This war in my mind overflowed to all aspects of my life. It was all-consuming and no one really knew. What you saw on the outside was not what was going on inside.

I mentioned what my war looked like, what does yours look like? Do you struggle with how you look? Do you feel self-conscious about your body? Do you and your bathroom scale scream at each other? Do you hate going to the doctor to hear about your weight-related health issues? Do you just want to feel attractive again? All these things lead us to feel like we are at war with ourselves. We want to do the right thing. We want to feel better. We want those jeans to fit perfectly, but we also don't want to give up all the things we love and think we can't live without. For me, it was fast food. I was a full-out, fast-food junkie. Even though I would do my best to eat healthily and follow the latest fad diet, in secret I was eating A LOT of fast food and I LOVED it! Food was my friend, food was my entertainment, and food was my comfort. I turned to food in happiness, sadness, and loneliness to shove down my feelings. I used food to numb my feelings. I often say food was my drug of choice. Maybe you can relate, maybe not.

At the age of 51, I had to start from scratch. I had a health crisis, and I knew that things had to change. I had to put aside everything I believed about my food and how to lose weight. I decided to follow a very structured program that would provide me with solid health habits and nutrition and help me drop the weight. What I learned very quickly is that eating smaller meals was key. I had eaten so little and gained weight that now eating six times a day was terrifying. I was confident it would never work for me. I was also confident that I could never be satisfied or content eating so few calories. So I was eating more than ever, but at lower calories. I increased my water and the scale started to move. Within days, I had trained my stomach and my brain that I was going to fuel my body often. For the first time, my stomach and brain were working with my body instead of against it. What I learned during this time was that trusting myself and listening to my body, basically eating along the lines of intuitive eating, had failed me because I had long lost trust in myself. Following a structured program helped me build trust in myself again. As the scale moved, I gained more confidence and then I really started digging into the reasons why I turned to food. I developed a far deeper relationship with pen and paper than I had with food. I spent every morning journaling, practicing, and spending time in my Bible. My faith has always played a huge role in my life, but there have been so many times that I felt ashamed and guilty over my eating and weight that at times I even tried to hide from God.

As the pounds continued to drop, I could tell there was a shift going on inside. I no longer felt like I couldn't resist temptations, my cravings disappeared, and what I craved was more of what I was experiencing. Having control over my cravings, food intake and emotions was priceless!

It was very difficult to explain how incredible and free I felt even while I was still in pain and dealing with complications and more back surgery. I pushed through, stayed accountable to my coach, God, and started living my life out loud.

In the past, sometimes weight loss terrified me more than weight gain. Anytime anyone would notice my weight loss or gain, I would immediately want to hide from the world. I would imagine their thoughts....

> Oh, she's gained weight AGAIN.
>
> She's lost weight... wonder how long that will last.
>
> She's so pretty, it's a shame she isn't skinnier.
>
> I wonder why she doesn't do something about her weight.
>
> I say I imagined these thoughts, but really what I was doing was replaying things in my mind that I had heard people say. My own thoughts were much worse.
>
> No wonder no one loves you.
>
> You will never succeed, you can't even stop eating.
>
> Nobody likes the fat girl.
>
> You look terrible, and no wonder things ended up the way it did.
>
> Your kids and family are embarrassed by you—this was the toughest one of all.
>
> Don't you know gluttony is a sin, how many times will God really forgive you?

I was so hard on myself, to the point I didn't even want to be seen. I was hiding in plain sight, but at the same time, I was mad at the world.

I felt lonely among many people. It was quite the mental war.

After losing more than fifty pounds, every time I tried to explain how I felt, all I could say was I felt like I had been set free from prison. I had a newfound freedom that really was freedom from my own mental war. When I started living my life out loud, sharing what I was doing to lose weight, it became easier and easier to accept myself as I was. I didn't put such high expectations on myself that I felt like I didn't measure up. I was having success and feeling great in my body and mind, and I finally started believing that saying…. If I'm still alive, God isn't done yet! I'm a perfect work in progress.

It was during this time that I felt strongly I needed to do a podcast. I had no idea how to do that, and I had no idea why anyone would want to listen, but it was a strong calling; so I did it. I spent six months writing, listening, planning, and learning from so many people. I'd get frustrated or stuck and I'd lay the podcast down. Then something would trigger me to start again. I almost named my podcast PRISONER OF WEIGHT but decided that if there was even a slight chance that would be offensive to any of our hard-working service members, it couldn't happen. I have the utmost respect for the sacrifice each and every service member and their families make to keep us safe, so I landed on *The War On Weight instead*.

On the podcast, I provide my listeners with resources to help them find freedom with food and motivation to treat themselves better and live as the healthiest versions of themselves, just like I did. I now find such joy in sharing my story and my struggles and providing women a place to come to armor up on their war on weight. I know God is using this podcast to heal my inner being, and it's setting other women free.

When it's time to go to battle with your weight, you need an army and a battle plan. Join me on the podcast to see if I might be the coach for you, or just armor up with some incredible resources.

And remember, IT IS NEVER TOO LATE to lose weight and feel great.

Philippians 1:6 NLT

And I am certain that God, who began the good work within you, will continue his work until it is finally finished on the day when Christ Jesus returns.

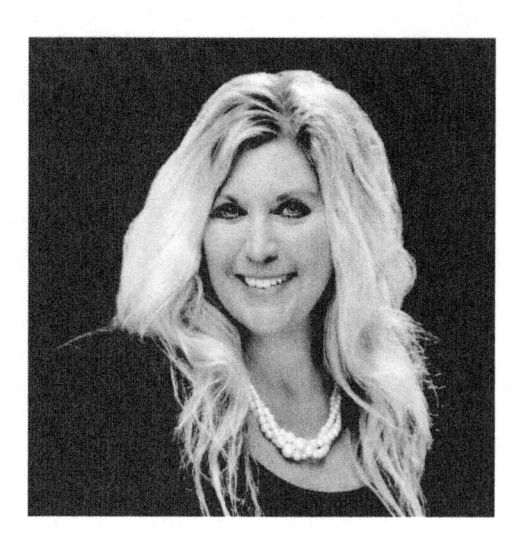

Pamela Kurt

Best Version of You, LLC
Professional Women Life Coach and Attorney

https://www.instagram.com/best_version_you/
https://www.facebook.com/bestversionyou
https://www.linkedin.com/in/pamela-kurt-41a26ba/
https://bestversionyou.com/
https://pamkurt.com/

Ms. Kurt is an attorney and business owner who has won many awards and honors, as well as held multiple leadership roles in her community. She owns Kurt Law Office, LLC with offices throughout northeast Ohio. She is also a best-selling author and public speaker. She has found a new passion. Her passion is to support and empower women to be the best they can!

The most personal enjoyment is when her clients find their own way. Ms. Kurt has a private professional women life coaching practice. BE THE BEST VERSION of YOU! This is an opportunity to elevate professional women to be the best version of themselves. Dream

Believe and Achieve is her signature coaching program. Her coaching program has allowed her clients on a powerful self-discovery journey. She is currently accepting new private coaching clients and is available for speaking engagements. Please contact her at BestVersionYou.com or PamKurt.com to start your journey to become the BEST YOU.

MINDSET IS THE KEY TO WELLNESS

By Pamela Kurt

"The key to a healthy life is having a healthy mind."
—Richard Davidson

As you start to think about wellness, it starts with your "mind." You start creating plans, ideas, and schedules, maybe even start researching food, exercise specifics, and more. It all starts with you being ready to start that journey. Let's set our mindset to be healthy, happy, and the best. Once our mind is set, we are on our way to health and wellness.

Mindset is EVERYTHING. Your mind can either make you sick or allow you to heal. I believe what you think affects your health. If you think you will, then you will, and if you think you won't, then you won't. "Your thoughts become things." You control whether you succeed, and it starts in the mind.

What is the wellness mindset?

The Well-Being Mindset is an awareness that health and well being exists.

- It's a mindset of having health and wellness that allows you to experience and live your best life.
- It allows you to care for yourself at a healthy level.
- It allows you to consistently pursue a healthy lifestyle.
- It means trying every day to care for yourself and be your best!

In setting our mindset we need to be aware of our physical, emotional, and spiritual self. We need to make ourselves a priority. YOU ARE IMPORTANT! You have heard the saying many times: before you can care for others, you have to care for yourself. How can you care for others if you have nothing left to give?

So many times us women wear many hats. We are everything for everyone. But you can't give away what you don't have. Treat yourself well enough to take care of yourself. Start with your mindset. The consequence of not caring for oneself can be devastating.

What are some of the things you can do to enforce your wellness mindset and put yourself forward?

1. *Get More Sleep* - The importance of sleep can't be overstated. The more rest the better we can be in all of our roles, and it helps with creative thinking and wellbeing. Try to get a minimum of six to eight hours a night. I know sometimes that isn't possible, but your health and mindset depends on the rest. More rest can also help us be better workers and support creativity. If you give yourself that time, you are on your way to being the best you.

2. *Reduce Stress* - This is a given. I know it's hard, but if something is causing you anxiety and stress, it's time to evaluate whether the thing or person causing you the stress needs to be in your life. Ever notice how after a crazy, stressful week at work you feel overwhelmed, rundown, and worn out? If you don't care for yourself, your body begins to break down. You get tired, headachy, grouchy, and less fun to be around. Stress combined with a lack of sleep can also potentially weaken your body's immune system, leaving you in a position of vulnerability for health-related issues. Even a few moments of solitude can make any day a bit better and help destress. You can also destress with meditation or try a hot bath – complete with candles, reading, or journaling. Turn off the TV and simply do things you enjoy.

3. *Let Relationships Thrive* - When you start taking care of yourself the people you care for the most will see a better, more rejuvenated you. By taking the necessary time for yourself, you give permission to your loved ones to take time for their own selves. Again, when you are well rested and relaxed you are more fun to be around. Soon, others will

notice you living with less stress and will want to follow your lead.

4 *Be kind to yourself* - Winston Churchill once said, "When there is no enemy within, the enemies outside cannot hurt you" and he was right; progress truly starts from within. Love yourself exactly where you are, right this moment, even if it's not "perfect" or you haven't achieved your desired weight or fitness state. Trust that you will reach your goals eventually, and remind yourself often.

5. *Find like-minded people* - Notice people in your life who enthusiastically support you and those who are doubtful of your lifestyle changes. Start by attending a wellness retreat. Wellness retreats are great places to make new positive-minded friends. Build your own supportive network.

6. *Be good to your body* - Much of our emotional state is related to our bodies, for better or for worse. Reduce feelings of guilt by eating properly and making healthy diet choices. Treat your body to soothing services at a holistic spa or massage center. Since mind and body are deeply intertwined, making changes to one is a useful way to ensure a shift in the other. Your body is there every morning for you, treat it well.

7. *Practice gratitude* - there is importance in feeling grateful, as it sets the stage for a positive mental attitude that initiates success in all areas of your life. Daily, write down a list of the things you're grateful for, even if it's simple. Sometimes we have to remember even the basics for our current health and abilities or even the roof over your head or a meal on your table.

8. *Consistency* - Find what works for you: daily, weekly, or monthly. Practice it and keep it going. Your body and mind will appreciate it and you will feel the difference. If you backslide into a negative mental pattern, don't worry. Simply replace the thought with something

positive. It does get easier over time. Journal some of your thoughts as you go through the process to see how far you have come.

9. *Have some fun* - When you are at your happiest, enjoy! Don't feel guilty for saying "no" to things that are important to you or you feel you don't need in your life. Find fun, and sometimes schedule fun time. It will be worth it. 10. *Pray-* Take time to have quiet moments with God. Sometimes it helps to pray out loud, alone in a favorite place, or even journaling your thoughts and prayers. Take the time for a spiritual connection to help with your mindset. Remember mindset and routine changes will not happen overnight. You've spent years developing specific mental habits, and it's unrealistic to expect that they will suddenly dissipate. But, when you actively begin to assess and improve mental patterns that might be holding you back, you'll find that all aspects of wellness start to get easier.

Remember, your wellness mindset is the starting point of your health and wellbeing. Wellness itself is a broad concept, a state of being where one's physical, emotional, intellectual, social, environmental, occupational, financial, and spiritual health are in balance and are supportive of a healthy lifestyle. When you value health and are motivated for quality of life potential, you will commit to positive behavioral changes and sustain a healthy lifestyle. You will become the best version of yourself with the help of your mindset.

Where is your current mindset? Do any of these look familiar?

Wellness Mindset	**Mindless Characterstics**
Grateful and giving	Not giving
Act Now	Procrastination
Evaluate problems with knowledge/tools	Blindly trust
	Accepting "whatever"
Trying new ways	Being pessimistic and negative
Being optimistic and passionate	
Doing it for my wellbeing	Being lazy and careless

Actively pursuing goals	Empty minded and passive
Focusing on actions/results	Focusing on failures
Analytical thinking	Reactive thinking
Peace	Anxiety
Freedom	Fear

When you are able to conquer your own negativity, overcome mental blocks, and master your mindset, you will make healthy commitments and be on your way to wellness success. With a wellness mindset, you will see your true values and fulfill your potential. You will make positive changes that align with your life goals. You will feel energetic and happy in your life.

If you are healthy and well, congratulations! But don't take it for granted Don't be afraid to start where you are. It is about progress and not perfection. No matter where you are, now is better than ever to make positive changes toward your wellness.

Where do you want to be? Don't sink into the busy work; it is common to get lost in life. Maybe you keep putting off wellness objectives just because you "don't feel like doing it." Do you want to feel life? Feel love? Enjoy the simple things? You can. Start taking care of your mindset. You just need to start! You don't need to be perfect, a certain weight, or have a certain income… You deserve to have the best life.

Most of our failures come from self-defeat. Take a step back. Sometimes, you are making your life choices subconsciously; you will be where you want to be or end up nowhere.

Life is limited, stop ignoring your health before damage is done. Healthy living is earned and no one can do it for you. You can do this. You can do it for YOU! You can be the best version of you!

I want to end with this.

A wise man tells his grandson: "there are two wolves in your head always fighting each other; one is a good wolf and another one is bad."

"Who wins?" asked the boy.

"The one you feed."

Feed the good wolf in your head and wellness will prevail. Use tools and develop a strong consistent path to a wellness mindset. You deserve it!

Be the best you as you head on your wellness journey.

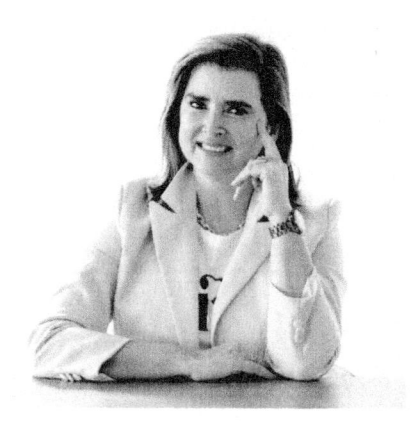

Paula Echeverri

CEO & Author

https://www.linkedin.com/in/paulaecheverri/
https://www.instagram.com/neuromomceo/
https://www.facebook.com/groups/505293884274103
www.neuromomceo.com

PAULA ECHEVERRI was born in Colombia, but spent half her life in the Silicon Valley in California where she started a family. She is a proud mom of two girls—9 and 12. She also worked with major companies in the tech space in Silicon Valley. She majored in advertising and also has a certificate in neuromarketing, applied neuroscience, and neuroscience for leadership.

After losing her hearing suddenly years ago with no apparent medical reasons from doctors, she did a lot of reading and research. She decided that there was more to life than limiting beliefs and that being stuck was not an option. The loss of her hearing triggered in her a change in her life, and how she perceived her reality, which helped her a lot in her path to heal herself and accept her new life using tools based on neuroscience.

YOUR MIND ON BEING YOU

By Paula Echeverri

It is the year 2048 and I wake up to live the best version of myself. I am living the life I was destined to live.

The world changed 10 years ago, and now everyone can turn their dreams into a reality. We discovered that now humans have the power to live the life of our dreams, and we woke to a new reality. Now everyone believes it is possible, and they know how to do it effortlessly and flawlessly through practice with the power of their minds. Illness is nonexistent, and biases disappear. All kids' schools changed the way they teach, and now they focus on brain power, neurology, and survival. Our new world defeated the old paradigm of fear and negative beliefs.

Do not Believe What Your Mind Tells You.

Hello, I am Paula Echeverri, and this is not the introduction of the next hit sci-fi movie. This could be a reality sooner than we think (or the beginning of my next book, so stay tuned!)

"We need to learn to live with the notion that our minds will try to sabotage us all the time!"

Let me explain why I wrote this title to start my chapter. Your mind likes things easy, and it will keep you within your comfort zone where there is no suffering, no change **and no evolution.**

So for lasting change, **we need to get out of that comfort zone.** It is important because if you have limiting beliefs like I used to have and negative thoughts from the past or fear of what could be wrong in the near future (what we call depression or anxiety), then your mental and physical health are at risk. Also, **when we struggle and change we**

build brain connections that are going to help us make better decisions in the long run.

I was living on the edge when I woke up having lost my hearing completely after having my second daughter. I was given no explanation as to why, since nobody in my family is deaf or has experienced hearing loss. I was born with normal hearing and lost it later in my life in my 40s when I was at the peak of my career in the Silicon Valley in California. I was completely shocked, as communication is so important. I was talking to investors and my team that I managed, so it was really difficult for me to understand why this happened to me.

We always take our senses for granted. After the initial shock, you try to find the why. I stayed there for a little, but what I needed was to accept my situation. That took me a little time, as I have always been independent and never needed help from anyone. So, accepting that I was now living a "life with limitations" was hard to endure.

We live in a reality that is all made up of our sensory experiences, such as our taste, touch, sight, smell, and hearing. I was used to having all my senses and losing one changed my reality and my perception of things.

I discovered later that I was flooded with a hormone called "cortisol," which is the stress hormone that the brain releases in a fight or flight response. Our fight or flight response is the natural alert system in our bodies that turns on when we have an emergency so we can survive. It is a primal instinct, but when we have it on for too long, it starts messing with our bodies. And guess what? I started feeling its effects after months of being like this. I was short of breath, had bad anxiety, fatigue, and a clouded mind, so it was harder and harder to function every day.

Our bodies are wise and they give us signals when there is a problem, but we ignore them due to fear or just not being able to accept our reality.

I had a panic attack and had to go to the emergency room. All the doctors checked on me, and they all said "you are fine"... I realized it was because my mind started producing all these problems in my body, so **I was not only deaf but also had symptoms that I created myself.**

I was poisoning my mind and body with my thoughts, and those thoughts made a huge mess in my body.

I decided from that day to take action and to be **ONLY the best version of myself.** I promised that I was going to cultivate my thoughts and my body for me, and my kids.

I read one book after another on the mind and body connection, I learned about neuroscience and became so obsessed that I finished multiple certifications. I started to crack the code on what was happening to me and my body. I felt more in control, but a little different after all the struggles. I EMERGED.

Emotions Don't Have to Be So Complicated, Right?

Wrong... I don't want to disappoint you, and yes, emotions are as complicated as a Mexican soap opera. I grew up in Colombia, and Latinos are very emotional and passionate, so I thought that was normal.

Looking at all the people around me being reactive and emotional in my family and our get-togethers (and living in what I now call a toxic environment) was the way I grew up, I was supposed to be an emotional, crazy Latina. It was culturally acceptable in my environment and when people were not like that, they were called stupid.

After many years of self-love and accepting my limitations, I realized I did not have to live like that.

It takes work to train the mind. It's a constant practice to reinforce new mindsets and to not live in the reactive state of the fight or flight response. Working at the root of why we created that problem in the first place and changing our perception of it by looking at different angles is key, too. We need to change the narrative and tell our mind a different story.

Many people have limiting beliefs in their subconscious mind and it's like "software" that needs to be deleted to make room for a new improved version. So, we need an antivirus to reset that system!

> Conscious Mind: Our thinking mind
> Subconscious Mind: Emotional mind.

Our nervous system needs to be in balance, and needs to center itself again after a problem, obstacle, or change in our life. That is possible by doing things to make it stronger and more in tune so you can bounce back faster from problems. That capability is called "resilience," and we all have it in us, some more or less than others, but we can develop this every day by going back to our senses.

We need to move from mindless to mindful, focusing and shifting attention to our senses. You are not your thoughts, look at them but don't judge them. That practice is called "Mindfulness." What we experience is based on our past experiences and sensory input, and we can control how we react to this.

Our brain is always making meaning out of everything we pay attention to.

So, if we focus on the positive, we will always get positive. But at the same time, if we focus on the negative we will get negative. Our health depends on our environment and thoughts.

We need a little toolkit of things that help us to regulate, so here are a few for when you start to feel triggered so that you can release happy feel-good hormones in your brain.

Try the following:

- Get a good hug (from somebody else or even yourself).
- Fake a smile (even if you don't want to).
- Notice that you're triggered. Say "I'm having an emotional reaction" or "I'm feeling triggered."
- Stomp your feet on the floor. Focus on the movement and the feeling of your feet.
- Take 1 to 1 five full breaths in one minute.
- Use a weighted blanket.
- A Cold shower or spray cold water on your face, or hold a cold bag of ice.
- Be grateful for something in your life.
- Pet a dog or an animal.
- Eat something sweet or sour.

If you do this consistently right when you notice you are getting triggered, you will reap the benefits in your nervous system and it will increase your resilience in the long term, which is what we need to have strong mental and physical health.

Only observing your emotions and never suppressing them is a way to regulate your nervous system with these tools. I also offer a great workshop on how to regulate emotions online because many people lack regulation and it requires practice. We mirror what our parents do, so if you had reactive parents who were not regulated you will likely become an unregulated adult.

You can be the writer of your own story, don't let life obstacles stop you. Instead, use them as motivation to build a strong foundation that you are proud of, we all can do it like i did.

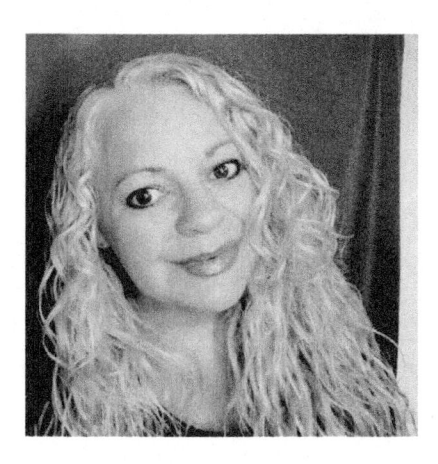

Heather Stokes Benton

Founder & CEO of Financial GPS / Financial GPS Mama
Podcast Host

https://www.linkedin.com/in/heather-stokes-benton-wealth-navigator-899624204
https://www.facebook.com/financiallyfocusedfamilies
https://open.spotify.com/show/7hb8W1oPbkv4UrgUz1ws9O?si=a5m-c4RyQpS6QF3JD Sqw

I am a wife, mother, homeschooler, and business owner. I am a giver, a motivator; a developer and I do not accept the answer no. I only see it as a challenge. My road to success has changed many times. Life has derailed my journey and I have built a new path each time. I went to college for Forensic Psychology and worked for multiple government agencies over the next eight years. When I met my husband he was a flight attendant and owned a limousine business.

We lived a lavish life. 9/11 was our first major setback, three years later he suffered a major injury and then pancreatic cancer at 40. I could have given up, but with three girls to depend on us that was not an option. I had to learn how to be creative with money. Now it is my mission to help others to go from surviving to thriving.

MONEY MADNESS & WEALTH HEALTH

By Heather Stokes Benton

We have heard them say in songs "I got mind on my money and money on my mind," and how sadly true that is. Several studies have demonstrated a cyclical link between financial worries and mental health problems such as depression, anxiety, and substance abuse. Financial problems adversely impact your mental health. The stress of debt or other financial issues leaves you feeling depressed. An individual's financial well-being is one of the greatest indicators of their mental wellness. A study published in 2011 by the peer-reviewed medical journal JAMA Psychiatry, compared the mental health of those making under $20,000 per year to those making over $70,000 per year. This research showed that low levels of household income are associated with several lifetime mental disorders and suicide attempts. The study also showed that a reduction in household income is associated with an increased risk of incident mental health disorders, substance abuse, and loss of sleep that can change physical health.

Is money significant? In short, yes! It is very important, and now more than ever given the economic landscape caused by Covid-19. Money is arguably the single most important construct for civilizing the modern world. The invention of money has established the consenting relationships between buyers and sellers, but also workers and owners. This medium of exchange is understood across the globe and is the foundation of our society. These small pieces of paper dictate almost every aspect of our lives; perhaps most importantly our mental health and stability. So, the questions are: How can we change our relationship with money? How can we start positive habits and rewrite our financial wellness?

Many people view money as dirty, negative, and even evil. I have found that most of the time these unhealthy views on money are because of generational trauma, historical standards, and gender inequality. What I found is that, for many of us, there is trauma associated with finances—trauma that has been carried through many generations.

We talk about the effects of historical trauma related to oppression and being marginalized. The intense emotions that come with financial struggles, however, are rarely mentioned. The shame, guilt, feelings of being gaslighted by your own bank account, memory loss about spending, paranoia that you were overcharged, and mistrust that you are underpaid are all part of the constant stress about money for so many women.

Women have increasingly become the sole provider for our households. We have obtained the highest rates of education and are progressively landing more management and leadership positions. Even in cases where men are the main household providers, women still play a vital role in making key decisions about how the money is spent.

However, there have been fierce and sudden changes in family structure caused by a history of patriarchy and white supremacy. Men continue to be torn from their families—lynched, imprisoned, and deported—leaving women to deal with the aftermath. Most women have never been taught to be confident with money.

There are so many subconscious ideas embedded in our relationship to money, generally tied to our sense of worth and value, and associated with crisis. Financial trauma is pervasive, yet largely unaddressed. The first step toward financial stability and wellness is identifying your relationship with money and what needs to change in your mindset. Understanding money is a tool we need to use, and it's within our control.

Let's shift gears and talk about controlling, managing, and growing our money so we can sleep at night, have less stress, and better overall wellness. I am going to give you a nine-step cure to money management to get you started on your path to financial wellness.

1. Get Organized: List all your fixed and variable expenses along with your debts (credit cards, mortgages, car loans, school loans, etc.) and any fixed or foreseeable expenses. Everyone's situation is different and there is no right way to organize your finances, but without some planning and organization, an unexpected expense can wreak havoc on a household that is merely gliding by paycheck to paycheck.

2. Track Your Spending: Keep note of what you're currently spending your money on. A $10 expense once a week may not seem very noticeable, but when you're spending over $500 a year, then you may determine that money is better being saved or paying off debt.

3. Stop Unnecessary Spending: Cut out frivolous spending where you can. If it isn't essential, chances are you don't need to have it. By working off a budget and tracking your expenses, you'll see how much you're paying for non-essential expenses, such as subscription services, ordering takeout, or entertainment purchases.

4. Live Frugally: Scale back on your flexible essential expenses and find ways to stretch how far your money goes. Here are some ideas: switch to a cheaper cell phone plan, downgrade your internet service, stop eating out and cook at home, choose generic over name brands, turn off lights and other electronics, and cancel subscription services you don't use often.

5. Set an Achievable Goal: Setting individual goals can help motivate you to save. Some different types of goals are creating

a budget, paying off debt, creating an emergency fund, saving for retirement or for a short-term goal, and building good credit. Defining and mapping out ways to achieve your goals makes reaching them easier.

6. Review Your Budget: Track your current expenses to get a clear view of the impact of inflation on your wallet. Some of the best apps designed to track your spending will also offer budgeting tools for free.

7. Spend Intentionally: If you don't need it, consider holding off on any new purchases until you can get the best deal. Wait until prices settle down to make big-ticket purchases, such as a new car or home improvement materials.

8. Be Flexible: Consider substituting used goods you can buy through online platforms or at thrift stores for non-food items like clothing, furniture, housewares, etc. Try eating at home instead of eating out. If you do eat out, drink water instead of colas, tea, or alcohol to save.

9. Change Your Habits: Consolidate errands and use public transportation when possible to use less gas. Use fans and open windows instead of turning on the air conditioning when it's hot and use blankets or layers to keep warm when it's cold before turning on the heat. To save on water, take shorter showers, and run full loads of laundry and dishes.

"Money can't buy happiness." Although it is cliche, it remains true. Being rich will not necessarily make you happier, but It will increase your standard of living and evaluation of life. What can help make an individual happy is making good financial decisions.

Your financial situation and mental health go hand-in-hand. If you can keep yourself from needlessly facing major financial issues, you are less likely to face mental health issues. I work with women and families every day to map out a new financial future for themselves and their family. Financial wellness is achievable. It does take intentional actions, but you can rewrite your financial path. I have had to rebuild several times in life which is why I help families go from surviving to thriving and building generational wealth.

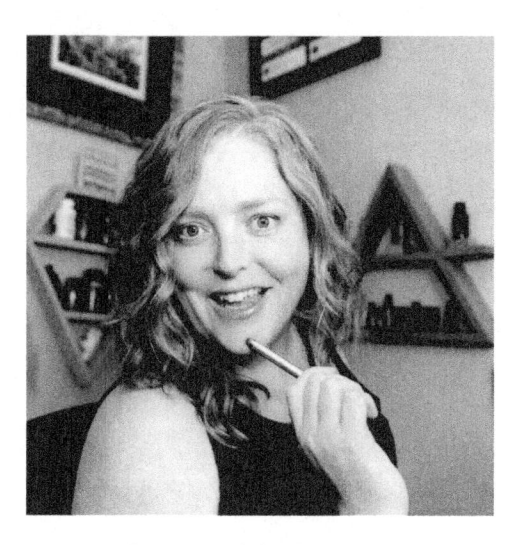

Colleen McCartney

Totally Essential Wellness
Holistic Tech & Wellness Coach

https://www.facebook.com/TotallyEssential
https://www.instagram.com/totally.essential
https://www.linkedin.com/company/totally-essential
https://colleenmccartney.com/
https://thewellnesscrm.com/

Born and raised in Northern Virginia with a heart for adventure, Colleen is a wife, dog mom, and aunt to nine tiny humans. Throughout her life she's been a medieval sword-fighting knight, mermaid trainer, cosplayer, Irish step-dancer, camogie keeper, health coach, and tech consultant.

She learned at age 14 that she was intersex, motivating her to become an advocate for herself and learn to care for this human body she was given. Lacking resources on this subject, she spent many hours at an old computer trying to make sense of it. That is, until she built her own computer, which inspired a lifelong passion for technology.

She loves sharing her story to empower people to make informed healthcare decisions for themselves. While her roots started in doTERRA, sharing plant-based solutions with others, she now runs Nerd Marketing Agency for entrepreneurs & agencies to get their businesses systemized, automated, & online.

BEING YOUR OWN ADVOCATE IN LIFE

By Colleen McCartney

At age 14 I was told I was a boy. I'd yet to start menstruating and went to see a (old & male) doctor about it. There was no softening of the news, just a simple statement that I had XY chromosomes and was, in fact, male. Just what every tall, ginger, freckled, self-conscious teenage girl wants to hear. It was at this point that I learned of a commonly expressed genetic trait in the females in my family that I had inherited. I had no idea this trait existed until this moment.

To say the least, that day had a huge impact on my life's trajectory. I realized then that I would have to be my own advocate because there was a severe lack of resources around the subject of intersex individuals. In trying to find healthcare providers, I've had varying experiences from straight-up refusal to treat me, treating me like a science experiment, tentatively treating me, and finally finding compassionate care. Heck, even my diagnosis has been renamed multiple times because there is still so much to learn about the human body. I felt like if a doctor couldn't help me manage my body, how in the world was I supposed to figure it out? I knew that if the so-called experts didn't have answers, I was going to have to figure things out for myself.

As I got older, I dealt with narcolepsy, chronic fatigue, anxiety, severe allergies, ADHD, and was on an emotional roller coaster due to hormone therapies. I gained a lot of weight from the hormones, and I was on medications to help manage my sleep and energy cycles.

Around the same time, I was working in the tech industry. The company I worked for had a chauvinistic, male-dominated atmosphere, and there were a lot of eyes on me as one of the only women in the office—the men got away with things that I couldn't, and it was a highly stressful and toxic environment. It provided a very good paycheck, but there was zero fulfillment or satisfaction in my life.

As a young adult, I was not healthy—physically or mentally—and didn't even realize how bad off I was.

Fortunately, a new friend shared doTERRA essential oils with me. I tried them and immediately felt relaxed, reaching a state of calm that I'd never experienced before. I legitimately wondered if these products were legal—I'd never had an experience with essential oils or anything else like this before. I was instantly hooked. I bought a small starter set, and after a week of consistent use and seeing the positive changes in my health, I turned around and bought one of their largest kits. I knew I'd finally found solutions for the health issues I'd struggled with my whole life, solutions I'd never heard of before, despite actively searching for something.

I was immediately drawn to the business side of doTERRA because I knew I had to get out of my toxic work environment. With this financial opportunity, I had the potential to not only create the life I wanted for myself but to make a positive impact on the world by helping other people find solutions to their health issues. Add in the fact that I could help other women leave the trappings of the corporate world, and it sounded like a great idea to me. I loved the idea of leveling up with other women and rising up together in business.

My team and I quickly found huge success sharing oils with people, and I leaned into my tech skills to make sure our customers were being supported systematically. But life has a funny way of teaching you lessons, and I ended up having to restructure my organization, which put us back at almost square one. I had to work through some trauma issues around the situation, and it took me a while to heal, get my head right, and refocus on my goals. But, I learned another important lesson by being my own advocate—even though I had to make a hard decision that affected me both personally and professionally, it helped me to identify negative relationships in my life and start to cut them out so I could be a healthier person overall.

As we grew and attracted new leaders, I shifted my focus to start looking for ways to support them. So many people would get excited about the oils' potential and want to share the amazing tools they had with everyone around them, but they would get overwhelmed with how to grow their business. They didn't feel like they could do what I was because they didn't understand the tech, and they weren't feeling successful. My tech and oil knowledge was intimidating to prospective leaders because they thought they needed to know as much as I did to be successful. But I knew that they just needed a few solid business tools and a simple strategy, so I went out looking for something that would help them grow their confidence.

I explored a lot of tech platforms hoping to find something that would have all the tools and functionality that my team needed to be successful. There were some promising options, but they required my level of tech skills, duct tape, and hope to keep them going, so we kept jumping from one thing to another.

Cue the pandemic, and I'd never been so happy to be surrounded by essential oils! At first, I loved quarantining because I had been putting everyone else's needs before my own for so long. I felt responsible for my team's downfall when we had to restructure and felt like I was always making up for it. I hadn't been taking great care of my health, and the pandemic was kind of like a reset for my entire life. Being at home gave me space to analyze self-sabotaging choices I'd been making.

Socializing was anxiety-producing for me, and I didn't realize it until my calendar was suddenly clear. I'd been holding on to some toxic relationships that I was finally able to let go.

I'd been making poor eating choices, and I adjusted my entire relationship with food. I began to look at food strictly as fuel and prepped my meals ahead of time so I didn't even have to think about what I would put in my body throughout the day.

I started moving my body daily, even if it was as simple as turning on music while working and having an impromptu solo dance party. I may have also thought—if the zombie apocalypse comes and I need to be able to run, I had better get my body in shape!

I started to recognize the intrusive (untrue!) thoughts that would initiate a catastrophizing hyperfixation, which would lead to spiraling self-doubt and crippling anxiety. I knew this pattern was affecting not only my professional life but my marriage and my relationships with my family and friends—and I just didn't feel like myself. There were many days when I would sit and think that the world might be better off without me in it. So, I now have a therapist in my life and am working on my relationships with myself and with my family.

Post-pandemic, I'm in a healthier mental and physical state than I have ever been.

I finally stumbled upon a customizable tech platform that would allow me to build the solution I'd been searching for for so long and have been able to share it with a wide range of wellness solutions providers who previously felt stuck in their businesses. I've grown my confidence to recognize that I can do amazing things and create solutions for people, and I know that I wouldn't have gotten to the point I'm at in life or business if I hadn't learned to be my own advocate. (My wild adventure in tech is a story all its own—check out the next book, Dream Big, Do Bigger.)

My experiences forced me to learn early on that I had to be the one in charge when it came to my health. I've always tried to bridge the gap between nature and science—I think there's a time and place for proactive self-care, and for modern medicine and pharmacological solutions. I am a firm believer that being informed about your body's needs and how all types of solutions work makes you the best advocate for yourself that you can be.

There's not much you can control in life. You control what you put in your body and how often you move it. You control whether you choose to share your needs with others and have honest communication. You are the one who occupies your body and mind and are the only person who can truly know what's going on inside it. At the end of the day, you are your best advocate—so stop doubting your awesomeness and second-guessing your intuition! Listen to yourself and reach for greatness!

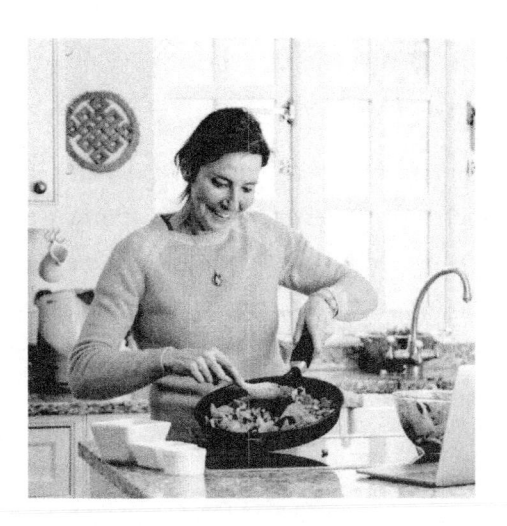

Catherine Rogers

Reset Your Health / Reset Your Brain Health,
reversing cognitive decline
Founder / Health Coach

https://www.linkedin.com/company/reset-your-health
https://www.facebook.com/resetyourhealthplan
https://www.instagram.com/resetyourhealthplan/
www.resetyourhealth.com
www.resetyourbrainhealth.com

Catherine Rogers worked in finance and the Guyanese jungles before becoming a mental health therapist and health coach passionate about the link between physical and mental health.

Trained in Neuro Linguistic Programming, Emotional Freedom Techniques, Cognitive Behavioural Therapy, and with a diploma in nutrition, Catherine provides a multi-disciplinary insight into health issues.

Her 20 years of experience and work with Oxford University PhD researchers looking at gut bacteria in relation to the immune system has led her to passionately believe in the importance of good gut health for mental and physical wellbeing.

This has led to her Amazon bestseller, "*Gut Well Soon*," which reveals how health problems are connected to gut health, Reset Your Health an online program providing recipes tailored to an individual's health challenges and food preferences, and Reset Your Brain Health, where she works alongside doctors to reverse dementia. All ground-breaking in the health space.

CALL ON DOCTORS BUT PLEASE ROW AWAY FROM MEDICATIONS

By Catherine Rogers

Let me share two health journeys with you, both with a 40+ year duration, to show you how crucial it is to keep away from the rocks of drug interventions, stay curious, avoid short-term solutions, and pay attention to lifestyle factors.

One is my miraculous recovery from migraines and the other is the incredible truth that dementia is reversible. Both involve calling on doctors but rowing away from drugs!

From the age of 14, I have had migraines. They have informed my behaviour, exam results, and many of my decisions.

I had migraines for 46 years—had being the operative word! No longer.

My migraines were painful but they were also the seeds that grew my Amazon bestseller, *Gut Well Soon*, which reveals how health problems are connected to gut health, and Reset Your Health, an online programme that provides recipes tailored to an individual's health challenges and food preferences. It also grew Reset Your Brain Health, where I work alongside doctors to reverse dementia.

I did everything—and I mean everything—to try and ease my migraines, including taking strong medications over 16 times in a single month to ease the pain. I changed my diet and removed inflammatory foods to reduce the frequency of the migraines. I also tried iridology, bioidentical hormones, avoiding alcohol, stretching, sleep pillows, magnesium supplements, and physiotherapy, and I have to say each thing helped me in its own way but did not stop the migraines.

I was told they were related to my monthly cycle (they are not), because

I clench and grind my teeth (I don't), get too stressed (not three times a week!), and that my sugar consumption was too high (I eat a low carb diet!). I tried Rolfing, Yoga, and meditation. Doctors told me migraines are, by their nature, multifactorial, but that they were unsure of the exact causes.

In 2020 I had a turning point. After years of physiotherapy which included stuffing lollipop sticks in my mouth to widen my jaw (which my surgeon subsequently said was a physical impossibility), I went to see a chiropractor. He came highly recommended firstly by my 75-year-old hairdresser Irene, who still regularly runs 10k, and secondly by my youngest daughter, Mia, a professional cricketer who is very demanding when it comes to quality of therapists. They both said he was very technically accurate.

After three sessions with chiropractor Kevin Woollett at KW Elite Chiropractic he said he would not continue to take my money until I had an MRI. He is a practitioner with total integrity. The MRI diagnosed a Wilkes 4 in both jaws.

What does this mean?

Well, my upper jaw is too small to allow my lower jaw to fit comfortably into it, thereby pushing it back, crowding my teeth and my entire lower jaw into a more backward and upwards position. This backwards compression of the lower jaw bone against the nerves, capillaries, and other soft-tissue elements within the jaw joint space damaged it over the years. The migraines have been caused by the resultant muscle tension around my scalp trying to defend the jaw for 46 years! Prescription drugs were my best friend.

So, now that I knew why I got migraines I was curious to find a solution. I found a dentist who proposed an appliance to allow my lower jaw to move down and forward and also to widen my upper jaw.

On December 9, 2020, I was initially given a hard, lower (occlusal) splint which stopped my migraines immediately. However I had no bite because the splint stopped my teeth from biting together and had to suck food, but it was worth it to have **no migraines**. I usually had three or four migraines a week, and while drugs enabled me to function daily, I hated taking them. The next step was orthodontic train tracks to widen my upper jaw and release the joint so I could attain a natural bite without impacting the jaw joint space. But progress slowed, and my amazing dentist, Caroline Bromley, at Ringley Park Dental Practice was frustrated. I was quite relaxed, as even though I had a mouth of metal I had no migraines.

I started to be curious about what could be stopping the jaw from shifting. I heard of a talented surgeon named Luke Cascarini who had started to put stem cells in the TMJ joint to help heal damage. However, this could only happen when sufficient space has been created, e.g. by a dentist to inject the stem cells into the joint. My jaw had moved a little, but not as much as expected by the end of 2021. In the intervening period, my surgeon recommended Botox in my jaw muscles to encourage the jaw muscles to relax.

Still no joy—the jaw would not budge. In January 2021 I visited the surgeon and had an MRI which showed the RHS jaw had space for stem cells, but the LHS had an adhesion. Everything was fused and no amount of physio with lollipop sticks or dental appliances and braces can shift a jaw that has fused. We decided to operate.

I had the surgery in April 2022. A camera was put into the joint and Dr. Cascarini was able to remove an adhesion on the LHS side with a two-way flush system. He flushed the joint and extracted stem cells from my hip marrow to inject into the joint so that the articular discs could regrow. Presto, onto the next stage of treatment and still no migraines! 😐 😐

I had to be careful with my jaw, eating only baby food whilst the stem cells took. No apple a day for me.

What does this journey show? For years, I rowed hard but continually hit the rocks of medications. Did I get lucky? Maybe, but I also had an open mind and kept looking for a solution. It was so worth it to be migraine free.

So, what of the other 40-year health journey? It starts with Dr. Dale Bredesen who, 40 years ago, was a researcher for big pharma hoping to find a drug that reversed dementia. He did not succeed, and to this day, despite billions spent by big government and big corporations, not one drug has been made that can reverse dementia. In fact, until now, dementia is considered to be both progressive and untreatable, but the Bredesen Protocol has proved otherwise.

Based on 40 years of research and pioneered by an internationally recognised expert in the mechanisms of neurodegenerative diseases, **<u>Dr. Dale Bredesen</u>**, the Bredesen Protocol has already reversed or inhibited the progression of Alzheimer's symptoms **in 90% of people treated**.

As of 2019 Dr. Bredesen has reversed 100 cases of dementia, and in his book, *The End of Alzheimer's*, he describes how to prevent and reverse the cognitive decline of dementia. I have one of the APOE genes which means that I am 30% more likely to get dementia. My father died with Alzheimer's, so they had my attention.

How does it work? Well, it is not drugs! The protocol focuses on addressing the root cause of Alzheimer's and the 36 contributory factors including nutrition, exercise, lifestyle, trophic support, and toxic loads. Dr. Dale Bredesen explains that Alzheimer's is a disease of both excess and insufficiency: excess sugar, excess toxins, low vitamin and mineral intake, low hormones, and lack of exercise. If addressing these does not improve cognition, he pushes his practitioners to dive deeper, looking at anything that might encourage the brain to create amyloid plaque as a defence mechanism. He stresses that the plaque that the drug companies have chased for years is not the cause, only the result. He has researched what prompts the brain to defend itself and once these prompts are removed, cognition improves and cognitive decline reverses. I have been a patient since 2019 and have seen fellow patients go back to work and re-recognise their grandchildren.

I am currently 30/30 on the MoCA score for cognitive abilities and follow the Bredesen Protocol (PreCode) as a preventive approach. Dr. Bredesen is passionate about people in their 40s having a "cognoscope," which is a simple blood test to work out their risk factors, and for people to remediate what needs remediating so they do not experience cognitive decline as they age.

Too often, Dr. Bredesen says people neglect their cognitive health until they have mild cognitive impairment, and they go to their doctors and are told: "it is just part of old age." When you get mild cognitive impairment, it has already been building for 20 years and is similar to metastasized cancer. But he is hopeful. Dr. Bredesen says "you have all met cancer survivors, but have you met dementia survivors? Well, you will now!"

Such an amazing journey of curiosity and rowing away from a drug solution. Bravo!

I am now a fully qualified Bredesen Apollo Health Coach working with the curious and talented Dr. Khelga Cooper Ivanova. I have no migraines or Alzheimer's, I am helping patients daily to reverse dementia at Reset Your Brain Health, and am currently writing an online resource to make the information more easily accessible.

My dream job was worth the 40 year wait. 😊

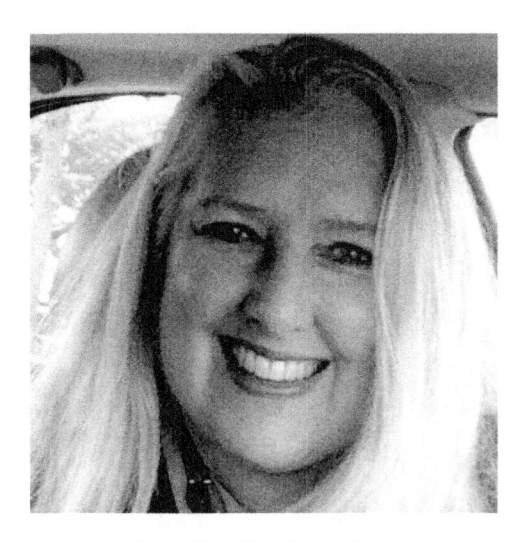

Dr. Shelby Decker

Shelby Decker Enterprises
Business Strategy Consultant, Coach. Veteran Advocate and Three Times International Best Seller Author

https://www.facebook.com/shelbymdecker
https://www.linkedin.com/in/shelbymdecker/
https://twitter.com/shelbymdecker
https://www.instagram.com/dr.shelbydecker/
www.shelbydecker.com

Dr. Shelby Decker Is known for turning ideas into profits specializing in business strategy, program development, and marketing. As a small business expert, she creates strategic programs. She puzzles together operations, communications, team building, and marketing for success. Dr. Shelby Decker uniquely creates initiatives meeting today's challenges for market gain. As a volunteer of a United Way of Broward County initiative, Mission United. Dr. Decker addresses veteran issues. Previous experience includes global corporations along with local and national non-profits. Dr. Shelby Decker attended Capella University for her Doctorate in Business Administration in the area of strategy and innovation. She earned her EMBA from the Jack Welch Management Institute, Strayer University. Bachelor of Science was gained at the Art Institute of Fort Lauderdale. She has a passion for helping others succeed with their goals with inspiration, empowerment, and education for increased community contribution. Visit http://www.shelbydecker.com to learn more.

OVERLOADED BUT NOT UNSTOPPABLE

By Dr. Shelby Decker

Yes, I Am One of Them!

The National Alliance of Caregiving (2020) reports 53 million of us are considered family caregivers. The report claims 61% of the family caregivers are female. There is little recognition, no tax deductions or salary for helping a family member as they enter into the new life phase of a disability or mental impairment. A family caregiver's average age is 49; 61% are employed, and 76% care for one adult. I am in the category of 24% who care for two or more care recipients. Yup, that's me! My mom is in a skilled nursing home, and my 86-year-old dad is my roommate. Like other 43 million caregivers, I do not get paid. I manage their banking, housing, monthly expenses, and medical needs. Dad adds the responsibility of daily engagement manager, transportation, and food buddy.

This is Crazy

What do you mean "No?" Dad asked.

"I have things to do," I replied.

"It takes a minute." He shot back.

I knew that he didn't understand. How did this happen? I yelled back in a parental voice, "I said no—why do you need an explanation? I can't do it now. My life can't revolve around you!"

Whoops—did I say that out loud? My heart rate and my blood pressure increased drastically. I can't do this anymore. My plan needs to accelerate. I need help. That night, with frustration and anger, I explained to my brother that I could not continue.

This is Not Working

Dad was taking up "my time," and not allowing me to address my career or nourish my life. I had all the warning signs of caregiver syndrome (where a caregiver needs time off and is away from caregiving responsibilities). I was avoiding my dad and suffering from exhaustion, depression, inadequate sleep, and irritability. I was frustrated!

My brother came for a visit. A month after, he was back to take care of Dad as I went out of town for business. The days away gave me what I needed to redefine my life. My brother was scared I would not return! He discovered the strain of being a caregiver. The conversations about dad shifted to how to get help to relieve the strain of caregiving for me.

Another month and there was another trip for my brother. We attended an out-of-town event that required us to travel by air, and my daughter helped with the navigation with dad. My brother took on some of the responsibilities of caring for dad during the trip. During this trip, my brother and I had many moments to discuss the next steps of getting help and each other's futures. We continued to discuss setting boundaries, reinforcing schedules, having non-caregiving activities, and having time for me. According to www.caregiver.com, caregiver recovery can take an estimated two years.

My brother is great at supporting me by listening without passing judgment and giving me advice. He came to the rescue to assist me at the time of burnout. Most importantly, my brother has given me accountability to change the situation.

How Did This Start?

For me, the caregiver role crept into my life. I was living with my parents as I was finishing my doctorate. My mother's health issues created a rollercoaster of emotional drama. My dad relied on me to do regular internet searches on her situation, drugs, and treatments. After a stressful weekend, my father realized we could not care for her at home and agreed to long-term care. The chore of addressing the necessary paperwork was a top priority.

Dad fell four weeks later, requiring 15 staples in the back of his head and nine stitches in the forehead. Immediately I became his driver to medical appointments. I was now going into medical visits to understand the necessary care for recovery. Then I noticed him forgetting things. Then there were more falls. A reverse shoulder replacement surgery resulting from a fall was required. More physical therapy visits were added to the list of doctors' appointments.

While all of this was happening, we moved. Added to the list of medical visits, I became a renovation project manager and estate cleanout services clearing 28 years of collections, clothing, and stuff. At this time, I took over the banking, automated most of the bills, and coordinated all the necessary transferring of utilities.

Getting Through It

It is not easy! Every caregiving situation is personal and unique. The care recipient's needs change every day. The process of memory loss could be slow over a while, and suddenly there can be a considerable decrease. at first, the caregiver can be straightforward with care. Checklists, schedules, planners, medical lists, medical records, and medicine lists are tools. Reaching out to services requires research of medical insurance provisions, local resources, and elderly programs. It can be exhausting and confusing. Address issues in chunks.

1. Form a team. Dad's doctor is terrific, and I count on him for many things. He understands dad's needs and listens to Dad and my concerns. He understands how one thing relates to another. I am beginning to rely on outside help in the transportation area. It has given me hours of freedom here and

there that quickly add up. My daughter has helped in little ways by checking up with dad, especially when I am out of town. Dad himself is a help. He communicates with mom daily and lets me know if she needs things. He is the one that brings things to her with his visits.

2. Create boundaries. It would be best if you value yourself as a patient as well as being a caregiver. Get someone who can be an accountability partner. Mine is my brother. He not only will step in if he can, but he has given me some harsh comments that keep me in check. It would help if you had someone who would be brutally honest and whom you respect.

3. An absolute must is that saying "NO" is okay. You can't feel guilty about sticking up for yourself. Dad has a problem with time management and commonly states, "it only takes a minute." That is true in his mind. You need to adapt and be proactive.

4. Keep your interests and add some. I learned you need five hobbies: physical, emotional, spiritual, financial, and growth. Currently, I am rearranging the content of these categories. I added yoga, and I am taking a speaking course. Make sure you continue with what nourishes your soul. Doing so helps nourish yourself and put up boundaries. Use appropriate coping methods like journaling, exercising, keeping your interests, and being with friends. I incorporate these every week. I schedule it. Yoga with a friend, daily calls to my brother, and continued participation with my passion for Veteran activities. It is easy to lose yourself, so I schedule it like a doctor's appointment for myself.

5. Recognize your limits. I wanted to be there for my parents, and I wanted to be the one to ensure they were getting the proper

care. It was tough for Dad to acknowledge that we could not give mom the proper care.

6. Make it fun and get them to participate. Dad always tells me which way the clouds are moving. I ask him about it if he doesn't comment. Dad loves to eat, so we go out often when he visits mom. We have our favorites, but we are trying new places. Dad likes sports, reading, and fitness. I am becoming more sensitive to getting him out and having fun. We are going to the farmer's market and having a game night (Chinese Checkers is one of his favorites).

Not Stopping!

I have been a caregiver for over four years. I feel blessed to be able to help my parents since they have helped me throughout the years. I did not sign up to be a caregiver and am not trained to be one. It is time for me to move away from the role of caregiving and become a daughter again. I am proud of what I have done for my parents, and I treasure our moments together. As I am writing this, I am shifting again to add help. Permit yourself to grieve. My relationship with my dad has been different since becoming a caregiver to him. It is okay to grieve about the past and honor those memories of that person while recognizing the person they are currently. Gain access to community resources. AARP has classes, the city has activities, and there is local senior care for daily outings. Dad is a Veteran, so I do an annual benefits checkup to ensure we are using his benefits. Being a caregiver has taught me many lessons. This new way of life is helping me define myself by being more assertive with boundaries, identifying my needs, and adjusting to the current situation while focusing on goals, health, and family.

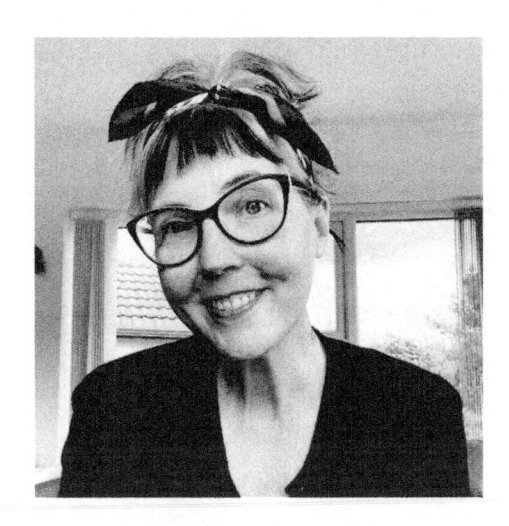

Jennifer Cairns

Founder of Rebel World, LTD and the Lady Rebel Club® movement

https://www.facebook.com/JenniferLCairns/
https://www.instagram.com/lady.rebel.club/
https://www.linkedin.com/in/jennifer-cairns/
https://www.ourrebelworld.com
https://www.ladyrebelclub.com

Jennifer's the Founder of Rebel World, LTD and the Lady Rebel Club® movement, where they empower, encourage, advocate for, connect and elevate women and all marginalized gender entrepreneurs who are neurodivergent or have disabilities.

Through Rebel World, she runs the Rebel Leader Institute, Rebel World Media, and Rebel Heart Publishing, which publishes the much-acclaimed book series Rebel With A Cause.

Being neurodivergent and having several disabilities, including Fibromyalgia, GAD, CPTSD, and rare blood cancer, Jennifer knows how high the hurdles can be for humans like her. Her heart, enthusiasm, passion, and grit show in everything she does.

She's an international bestselling author, brand and business mentor, neurodiversity and disability advocate and self-empowerment speaker.

Jennifer lives in N. Ireland with her husband, two boys, and their dog. She believes with her whole heart we all have value to give and that being different doesn't mean less.

REBEL HEART

By Jennifer Cairns

I have a rebel heart, and often we need to make sure that we use our rebel hearts to love ourselves just as much as others. Loving ourselves means taking care of ourselves. Ironically most rebels I know (myself included) aren't always great at putting themselves first. This is why following what I call a *Be More Rebel*™ self-care strategy is important. And it takes guts to implement.

This isn't something I started to put into practice overnight. My long-term journey with undiagnosed neurodivergence, anxiety and mental health disorders, and other disabilities has taken its toll. I self-medicated, self-harmed, and had a chaotic lifestyle for many years before marrying my husband now of 21 years. When you're "different" or suffer any kind of trauma or neglect—you're rebel heart often blossoms with the determination to improve things for others and overflows with empathy.

Yet, it's taken a very long time for me to put myself in the "needs attention" pile. And some days/weeks, I still don't. I find this is something that takes constant work. Yet the more messy and chaotic my life gets, the clearer I've seen where so many humans like me fall into this trap and how they carry around the shame others have placed on us. I'm now better equipped with the strength and tools to not only better support myself and my family but my business, and others, too.

REBELS HAVE G.U.T.S.

Being a rebel means that we often defy the odds and do hard stuff every day. We need to open up our rebel hearts, embrace ourselves, and have the G.U.T.S. to care for ourselves like we need to. What happens when we don't? Our illnesses, conditions, disorders, and how our neurodiversity impacts us all compound. Stress exacerbates all of these things, and hiding those parts of us away or not taking care of ourselves like we should cause us huge amounts of stress. Yet, if we have G.U.T.S. we can get off that hamster wheel and likely improve our life, relationships, businesses, and impact.

G.U.T.S. is an anagram for grace, understanding, treat, and stop.

GRACE

This could be an entire book series. We can give grace to many of those around us—when they miss a meeting, are off ill, or struggle to cope for any reason. We can even be the first ones to jump in and help! We'll take on more and give more, yet when we need help, we fail to give ourselves the grace to not only be ill but also when we need space, recover, or slow down.

Forgive yourself for all the times up to this point that you were late, missed a deadline, didn't finish a project, lost that third set of car keys, drifted off during a chat with your biz bestie, or didn't reach those goals. Forgive yourself for being hard on yourself. This again is especially a hard one for me and I struggle with giving myself grace a lot of the time.

Give yourself room to mess up. We must test them, tweak them, fail, and improve them. Yet, we can often take these as our failings, and they're not. They're part of growing a business, and if you permit yourself to mess up, you'll find it easier to learn from those mistakes and see them as opportunities.

Giving others and ourselves grace isn't weak. It is a strength. Here are some ideas to think about:

- If you have a daily routine, incorporate grace into it.
- Make a list of unique things you've accomplished daily, week,

- Say one grace mantra each day. Mantras are great to help shift or reframe a thought or mindset. You could have ones like "I am not my mistakes," "I refuse to apologise for being me," and "I am enough." If you are stuck on a specific negative thought and need some help to overcome it—write a mantra to help you support and reframe it.
- Give others grace. For many of us, it can be difficult to give others grace about specific things, too. The more we can understand that nobody is perfect, that we all make mistakes and imperfections, the easier it is to give ourselves grace.

month, quarter, or year. Build this into your routine, too.

Giving yourself grace is a marathon and not a sprint. You should build into your routine slowly so you're more likely to stick with them. Some of this self-care may not initially feel overly comfy for us. It doesn't always work for me, but slowly I've gotten better at it, and so can you.

UNDERSTAND

Most of us, especially those with rebel hearts, tend to be empathetic and understanding with others. Ironically, being understanding with ourselves isn't as easy. We are often so driven to be there for others, support others, and make that big impact that 'we' don't even think about how we are getting all of the things done that we do. We push ourselves into overdrive and often into burnout. Understanding ourselves better can help stop that from happening.

Understanding how you function best by learning what your current limitations, triggers, weaknesses, and strengths are will significantly help you in your life and your business. You need to do the work to get to know yourself better.

- How good are you at using words or images to alter your feelings about a situation, person, task, or even yourself? What

works best for you—reading, visualising, or listening? We all like and even process things in different ways.
- How long can your work on or do something before losing focus or energy?
- Are you better at pacing yourself over a more extended period, or are you better at working at a higher pace and capacity in shorter bursts? Knowing this can help you better plan your day.
- Are you a morning person or an evening one?

For many of us, understanding how doing XYZ will affect us is key, as we can then plan. Will that trip to the zoo push you past your capacity for the day? If so, will it take you one day, three days, or even a week to fully recover? If you have some idea for these things, you'll be better able to plan and prepare for those days that come in the aftermath.

TREAT

We all need to treat ourselves occasionally. It's a proven form of self-care, yet many of us either treat ourselves too much in the wrong way (yes, eating ice cream for dinner every week falls into this category) or don't treat ourselves at all.

Dopamine shortages can affect and impact our focus, mood, motivation, attention, and even how impulsive we feel at any given time. There are natural and easy ways to provide a little dopamine treatment. Find what works well for you and your life. There's no point in telling you to jog if you have a medical condition or disability that prevents you from doing that. Yet finding your dopamine rush from that tub of ice cream for dinner isn't doing you any good either.

A treat doesn't have to be food or expensive. For me, a treat is walking by the coast with a nice cuppa. I love the sea, and don't mind bundling up for fresh sea air. The important thing is to build these into your day. Think of your treat like your oxygen mask. Put yours on first to ensure you're well enough to do all the amazing things that you want to do.

STOP

Let's face it; we are often queens of stressing the little things, big things, and all the in-between. Our often-strong empathy can make us concerned for society, climate, nature, friends... the list goes on. So, what can we do?

We need to find a way to still be "rebels" yet not allow ourselves to become overwhelmed by all of the many things we're driven to fix, change, or do.

Stop apologising, blaming, and beating yourself up. Stop allowing others to blame you for everything, too. I took the blame for everything for so many years and it wore me down. Let's drop that shame and disappointment and accept that we're not perfect but also not responsible for everything that has happened or will happen in the future.

Have guts and give yourself and your rebel heart the time, patience, understanding, grace, care, support, and love you need. Being more rebellious in this way creates plans, a business, self-care strategies, and even a life that suits you and makes you happier, healthier, and better able to do all of the things and have the impact that you want. It isn't selfish to *Be More Rebel*™ with your self-care, it's allowing you to better fuel your mind, heart, and soul.

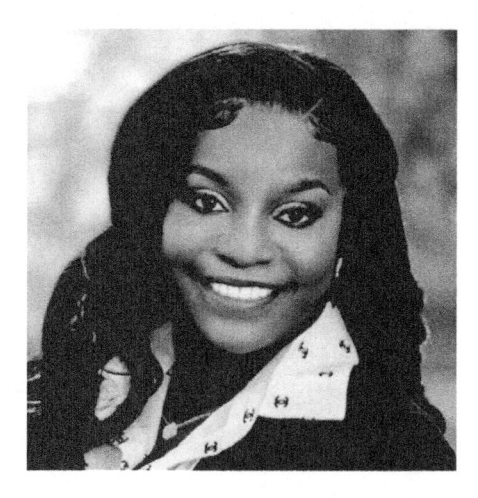

Lovely LaGuerre

Founder & Owner of Pure Heavenly Hair and Beauty

https://www.instagram.com/PureHeavenlyHair/
https://www.instagram.com/LovelyVegasCommercialLV/
https://instagram.com/pureheavenlyhair?igshid=YmMyMTA2M2Y=
https://www.facebook.com/pureheavenlyhairboutique
www.PureHeavenlyHair.com
www.LovelyInspireYou.com
www.LovelySellsVegas.com

My goal is not to be better than anyone else, but to be better than I used to be.

Lovely LaGuerre is a successful Commercial and Luxury Real Estate Agent, founder of Pure Heavenly Hair Boutique, and author who has always enjoyed a passion for supporting and empowering other women. She believes that, by working together and harnessing the power they share, women can become unstoppable forces, leveraging their potential and giving back to their communities.

As a serial entrepreneur and a wealth creator to others, Lovely also writes her own books and has contributed to others as well, including

The Successful Woman's Mindset: 21 Journeys to Success and Becoming an Unstoppable Woman.

In her latest offering, *Becoming an Unstoppable Woman Entrepreneur*, she shares empowering, inspiring, and uplifting stories that are designed to help women to succeed. This is to be followed by *Becoming an Unstoppable Woman in Finance, Unleash Her* Book, and many more.

In her free time, Lovely enjoys traveling, good coffee, reading, and meditating. She is also someone who is determined to give back to the community wherever possible and make a difference in the lives of others. As such she regularly volunteers in local communities. She is a member of CALV, NAR, LVR Association, and many more.

THE WEALTHY MINDSET AND WELLNESS: A HOLISTIC APPROACH TO HEALTH AND WELLNESS

By Lovely LaGuerre

INTRODUCTION

LOVELY LAGUERRE IS A WEALTH CREATOR. AMAZON BEST SELLING AUTHOR. A COMMERCIAL AND LUXURY REAL ESTATE AGENT. SHE IS ON A MISSION TO HELP OTHERS TO TURN THEIR REAL ESTATE INVESTMENT DREAMS INTO A REALITY. SHE IS ALSO THE FOUNDER OF PURE HEAVENLY HAIR AND BEAUTY BOUTIQUE, A LUXURY BEAUTY BRAND THAT WILL TRANSFORM, INSPIRE, AND EMPOWER ANYONE TO UNLEASH THEIR BEAUTY FROM INSIDE. SHE IS A MEMBER OF CALV, NAR, AND LVR ASSOCIATION, AND MANY MORE.

It is no secret that a small minority holds the vast majority of wealth in our society. What is less well known, however, is the fact that this disparity is also reflected in our health and well-being. Generally, those with more money can afford better healthcare, have more access to healthy food and lifestyles, and enjoy greater psychological and physical well-being than those less well-off.

I am here to share that when you aim and take a holistic approach to your health and wellness, taking into account not only the physical aspects of health but also the mental and emotional dimensions, the journey can be tremendous. We will explore how our thoughts, emotions, and beliefs can impact physical health and learn how to use positive thinking and self-care to improve overall well-being.

So, if you're ready to take your health and well-being to the next level, this book is for you! Let's get started!

THE WEALTHY MINDSET

Your health and wellness are not just about physical health. Taking a holistic approach that includes your mind, body, and soul is essential. This means that you should focus on your overall well-being and not just on one aspect of it. For example, you should not just focus on your physical health but also on your mental and emotional health.

This approach to wellness is important because it can help you achieve balance in your life. When you're in balance, you're better able to manage stress and stay healthy. Additionally, this approach can help you feel more connected to yourself and others.

Having a Wealthy Mindset is all about inviting abundance into your life. When you have an abundant mentality, you believe there is enough for everyone. You think big and go after your dreams. You understand that you are worthy of love and success.

The idea that only people with millions of dollars in their bank accounts qualify as "rich" may be the most significant wealth myth. Nothing is falser than it is today. Anyone can have a wealthy mindset—regardless of their income.

So, what is the wealthy mindset? It's about having an abundant way of thinking and attracting wealth into your life. It's about thinking big, going after your dreams, standing in your power, and knowing that you are worthy of achieving success. Most importantly, it's about taking care of yourself first.

When you have a prosperous mindset, you realize there is enough for everyone. You don't feel resentful of others' success because you understand there is plenty of room for everyone to achieve their goals. Instead, you focus on your journey and trust that everything will work out in the end by believing in the process.

The wealthy mindset is also about being generous with your time, energy, and resources. When you're generous, you attract more affluence into your life. Giving creates a state of abundance, which in turn attracts more abundance. It's a cycle that starts with you and begins with your mindset.

If you want to achieve balance and success in your life, start by changing your mindset. Adopt a wealthy mindset and watch as your life transforms for the better.

What are some ways that you can adopt a wealthy mindset?

- Think big and go after your dreams
- Understand that you are worthy of love and success
- Prioritize taking care of yourself first
- Have an abundant mentality
- Focus on your journey
- Be generous with your time, energy, and resources

Start by changing your mindset and watch as your life transforms for the better. Adopt a wealthy mindset today!

YOUR HEALTH IS YOUR WEALTH

If you're thinking about your health and well-being from a place of abundance and prosperity, you're already on the right track. A wealth mindset is about believing that you deserve good things, including a healthy body and mind.

When it comes to your physical health, a rich mindset can help you make choices that align with your goals. For example, if you believe you deserve to be healthy and prosperous, you're more likely to make choices that support those beliefs. That might mean eating nutritious foods, exercising regularly, and getting enough sleep.

It's also important to remember that your mental and emotional health is just as important as your physical health. If you're feeling stressed, anxious, or down, taking care of yourself emotionally is essential. This might mean taking time for yourself, practicing self-care, or reaching out to a therapist or counselor.

A healthy mind is a wealthy mindset. By taking steps that support your well-being, you can create a life that is abundant in every way.

By making these changes, you'll see a real difference in your physical health and overall well-being. You'll feel happier, more confident, and more able to care for yourself physically and emotionally. So if you're ready to change your life, start by changing your mindset!

WHY IS A HOLISTIC APPROACH TO HEALTH IMPORTANT?

A holistic approach to health is necessary to address the issue's root rather than merely the symptoms. It considers all factors and motivates individuals to care for their health and well-being.

Finding long-term treatments for current disorders and preventing new ones are equally important. For instance, drinking caffeine or energy drinks can be the first thing you do if you are feeling low on energy. This might only be a temporary fix. But an illness may be underlying, and the lack of energy may be a sign. When considering all facets of holistic health, it is possible that anxiety, sadness, lack of sleep, low testosterone levels, and even diabetes are to blame for a person's lack of energy. Evaluating holistically is the goal.

HOW CAN YOU LEAD A HOLISTIC LIFE?

Having the mentality that the few aspects of your health can be considered for you to function at your best is the first step in adopting a holistic way of life.

You can create an integrated lifestyle in addition to adopting a holistic diet by doing the following:

MEDITATION

Meditation must train the mind to develop lasting mental clarity, equilibrium, and mindfulness. It has been demonstrated to be a valuable method for controlling stress, anxiety, and depression and fostering general well-being. Even 15 minutes of meditation can help you become calmer and more focused while also helping you manage emotions better.

SLEEP

The time of day when you can physically and psychologically refresh is when you sleep. Maintain a regular sleep schedule, abstain from alcohol use and big meals in the evening, and avoid naps during the day.

I can relate, stressful situations and events and regular sleep pattern disruption can all lead to temporary sleeplessness. On the other hand, underlying medical conditions like aging, drug side effects, anxiety, and mental health issues can all contribute to chronic insomnia. Although it could be a better option than sleeping drugs, a holistic approach supports addressing the root of the problem. Please find the underlying causes with your doctor's help so they can be treated.

PRACTICE INTUITIVE EATING

Intuitive eating promotes a positive relationship with food by relying on your body to make the best decisions rather than following diet fads that impose time and food restrictions. An intuitive eater follows this method, mostly eating when you are hungry and stopping when you are full. This is accomplished by being adept at identifying emotional hunger apart from physical need.

The body will convey signals such as a growling stomach, irritation, and exhaustion to replenish nutrients for energy consumption. In contrast, emotional need brought on by boredom, loneliness, and misery causes emotional hunger, which causes cravings and overeating.

Studies show that intuitive eating can be a comprehensive strategy for managing weight, blood pressure, and much more.

BE ACTIVE

With numerous advantages, including a lower risk of heart disease, stroke, type 2 diabetes, and various malignancies, physical activity may be one of the most affordable ways to enhance general health. Exercise has been demonstrated to increase mood, self-esteem, and sleep quality while lowering the risk of stress, depression, Alzheimer's disease, and dementia.

The National Health Service recommends that adults exercise daily to complete at least 150 minutes of physical activity per week.

Having a holistic outlook on life entails caring for every facet of Who You Are. Your ability to benefit most from your health and well-being will increase as you embrace a more integrated lifestyle.

CONCLUSION

There is a disconnect between the way we are taught to think about our health and well-being and the way we experience it. The good news is that changing our mindset and creating a more holistic approach to health and wellness is possible. By connecting with our inner wisdom, listening to our bodies, and making self-care a priority, we can close the gap between our current reality and our desired state of health and well-being. Wealthy Mindset and Wellness offers readers the tools they need to make this shift in thinking, providing them with an actionable framework for creating lasting change.

I hope this book will be a valuable resource for women or anyone who are ready to make their health and well-being a priority. Thank you for taking the time to read it. I hope you find the information inside helpful and empowering.

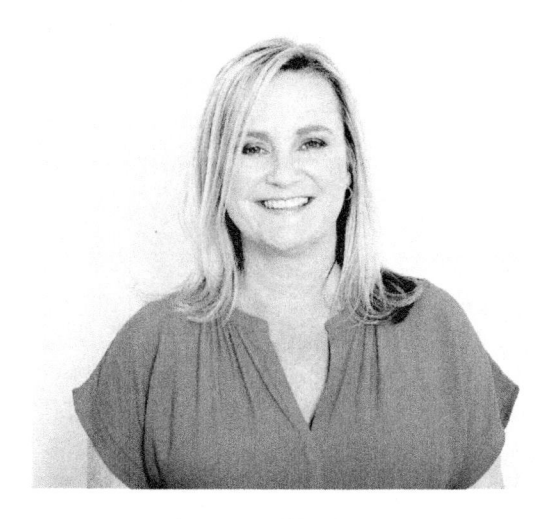

Natalie Pickett

Entrepreneur, Founder and CEO of Wellness on Time

https://www.linkedin.com/in/natalie-pickett-74b00910/
https://www.facebook.com/wellnessontime/
https://www.instagram.com/natalie_Pickett_Mentor/
http://www.nataliepickettmentor.com/
https://www.wellnessontime.net/

Natalie Pickett is an award-winning business leader and sought-after mentor and speaker. A best-selling author, Natalie has been featured in major publications including *Authority Magazine*, Ariana Huffington's *Thrive Global and Entrepreneur*. Natalie started her entrepreneurial career 30 years ago, and is founder of multiple businesses, with 6 and 7 figure success stories. She says "Success is less about hard work and more about finding joy in your every day." Utilizing her business, fitness, and tourism expertise, Natalie created Wellness on Time, a publisher and online wellness program. As a former fitness instructor, when ill or injured, Natalie sought activities for recovery with less ongoing therapy and greater ease of movement. "Finding ways to reduce stress and enhance your body movement can bring health benefits and greater life enjoyment."

Wellness on Time helps people to easily integrate wellness activities into their every day through books, magazines and the 28 Days of Wellness program.

LIVING THE DREAM THROUGH WELLNESS

By Natalie Pickett

What an experience becoming an international best-selling author in the *Becoming an Unstoppable Woman* series has been! My previous chapters focused on "Living the Dream"—and while everyone wants to live their dream life, what does that mean to those for whom it may seem out of reach?

Wellness is key—when we don't feel well, we feel poor, and our health is our wealth. It's hard to feel good when we don't feel well, and the key to feeling good and living our dream life is following our joy. How do we get to the place where we have those moments of "Living the Dream," and feel like we are living our best lives?

I have always lived an active and healthy lifestyle. Raised by a "hippy" mother, we ate whole foods, grew our own veggies, and went to hippy communes for school holidays.

In my early twenties, I became a fitness instructor and travelled the world before transitioning into the tourism industry (starting as a tour leader in Europe), before moving back to Melbourne and starting my inbound travel company bringing international tourists to Australia.

Over the years, my health issues have included: injuries from a car accident; quarantine in London due to an unrecognisable parasite from a trip to Egypt(!); pelvic instability (overstretching of the ligaments due to the *relaxin* hormone, causing chronic pain due to all of the surrounding muscles in constant contraction trying to hold you in place) during pregnancy and years afterwards; a freak accident with a fit ball bursting and dropping me onto a tile floor causing a damaged coccyx; abdominal separation (*diastasis recti*) that possibly occurred during pregnancy but was diagnosed years later; and recently, a broken leg from a hiking accident, that required two surgeries and left me enduring years of chronic pain.

It's a bit of a list, but none of it is terminal and we all have issues—some we can manage ourselves and others that we need help managing.

Although I have always been fit and active, there are times when I needed to adapt—even if just for the short-term.

14 years ago, everything around me collapsed. My husband and I separated, and my travel business I had worked so hard to create and grow for 15 years had to close due to the global recession. Getting through my days was painful, but I searched for ways to support myself—different therapies, energetic healings, breathworks, meditation, and traditional therapy. I learnt that so much healing can be achieved through meditation and tapping into our intuition to understand how our body is feeling and understand what needs to be healed. In one breathworks session, in a deep state of supervised meditation, I felt my shoulder being moved and adjusted. I wasn't consciously moving it and no one was touching me, but my shoulder was moved (like a chiropractic adjustment) back into place and the pain was gone! Our bodies have a great capacity to help us heal, and the more I investigate, understand, and listen to how I'm feeling, I am constantly amazed!

While our bodies are designed to handle small doses of mental or emotional stress, we are not equipped to handle chronic stress without consequences.

Chronic stress can come from finances, deadlines, expectations, workloads, living in unsafe conditions, or concern for the wellbeing of loved ones. The experience of chronic stress causes increased heart rates, breathing to quicken, muscles to tighten, and blood pressure to rise.

Most symptoms of chronic stress are physical—headaches, stomach aches, digestive issues, muscle tension or pain, sleep problems, chest pain, fatigue, changes in sex drive, and it can cause weight loss or weight gain. Stress also causes an increase in the hormone cortisol, which researchers have linked to serious health issues.

Therapy for our emotional wellbeing, combined with physical therapies for our bodies, can make a huge difference. In recovery from injuries, I had chiropractic adjustments and did Pilates regularly. While I appreciated this support, I became curious about how my physical health could be improved without needing regular therapy. Discovering Feldenkrais was a mind-blowing experience! In my career as a speaker and mentor for personal and business development, I often talk about patterns and how the extremely strong emotional patterns we have formed result in often repeated behaviours that may not be serving us well. Likewise, with our body, we have formed pathways from the brain that have formed patterns of how we do a particular movement. For example, once you established how to move your body in a certain way, like moving your right arm forward, a pathway was formed in your brain to imprint this, like a habit—and every time you move your right arm forward your brain moves it the same way. If the way you are moving is causing problems, you will continue to perpetuate this pain until you change the habit. Named after founder Moshe Feldenkrais, Feldenkrais (also known as Awareness Through Movement), is a series of small movements with no stretching whatsoever, showing your brain there is more than one way to do the movement. By exploring these movements you can release and change your range of movement substantially. Incredibly, I had an injury release in one group session, with no massage or manipulation, no stretching, no pain, just release. Our bodies are amazing, and once we are aware of how we use our bodies we can take responsibility for healing and manage this to take better care of ourselves. Not "pushing through the pain," but understanding the pain and making your body movement easier.

Learning to love and support our bodies is as important as supporting ourselves emotionally—and the quickest way to make this change is by being kind to ourselves. After one energy healing session, the healer told me: "It is like you have been beaten up, but I think you've been beating yourself up." She was right. My inner voice was my inner critic, and this pattern was something imprinted from childhood. "Our inner voice should say things that we would want our very best friend to say."

It's important to find ways to accept responsibility for our wellbeing and look after ourselves. We all want to be healthy, but stress, time restraints, and a lack of knowledge about what to do are preventing people from being active. In 2014, I launched "Wellness on Time", an online wellness program featuring a range of modalities such as Yoga, Pilates, Tai Chi, Circuit, Meditation, and, of course, Feldenkrais. It has short classes that can be scheduled into a busy day. "Make it Easy, Make it Fun" is one of our mottos. No one should spend their days on a diet or exercise program they don't enjoy!

The keys to success with each of my businesses are that they come from my passion, my core values, and my desire to share my knowledge with others. When things become stressful, your values will drive you! By taking positive steps for your wellness, it is possible to define your version of success and take the necessary steps to achieve your goals. Explore different activities and choose those that bring joy.

Here are my top tips for integrating wellness into your everyday.

1. **Make it a priority.** Say it to yourself, say it to others: "My health and wellness are important to me!" Diary it first and don't concede that time for other appointments.

2. **Don't try to do it all at once.** If the changes are too severe,

you may find it difficult to sustain. Rather than trying to change your whole lifestyle overnight, start with a small change and integrate that first.

3. **You don't have to be perfect.** Nothing makes us feel like quitting more than when we turn up for a group workout and we're struggling while everyone else seems to be brilliant at it! It is not a competition. Take small steps to improve your technique or efforts each time.

4. **Be your own best friend**. Be aware of your self-talk. Calling yourself a loser will have a devastating effect. Be your own support person, and acknowledge that you are improving even if it is just by turning up.

5. **Feeling good.** Changing to achieve healthy habits is not an end goal, as your life is ever-evolving. It is a process, a lifestyle choice. If you make changing the habit the goal, then what will you do when you reach your ideal weight or body shape? You might stop. Embrace the process and enjoy the activities so that enjoyment and benefits of feeling good as you make improvements become the reward.

6. **Get started today.** Small steps can make a big difference. We can easily find reasons for not starting—busy, tired, need new workout gear, etc. Take a small step to get started today!

You can find more details about Wellness on Time on the links in my bio.

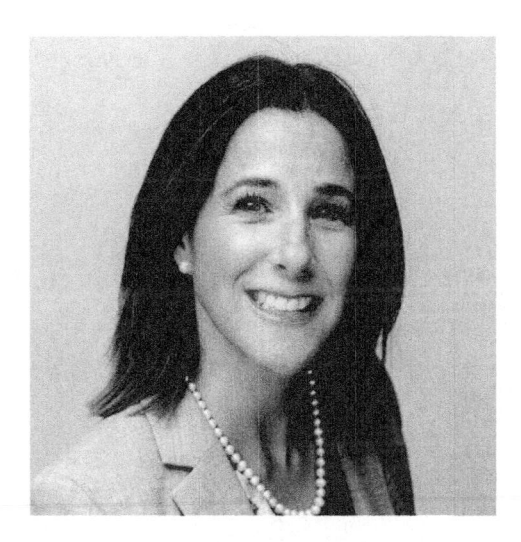

Michele Kline

President & Founder of Kline Hospitality Consulting LLC

https://www.linkedin.com/in/michelekline/
https://www.facebook.com/klinehospitalityconsulting
https://www.instagram.com/michelekhnecoaching/
https://www.klinehospitality.com/
https://www.klinehospitality.com/services

With intentionality and dedication, Argentinean immigrant Michèle Kline, built a career in the Hospitality Industry "playing chess and not checkers."

In 2010, she founded "Kline Hospitality Consulting," where she enhances companies' culture and improves their operating procedures, with laser focus on leadership development. In 2018 she received the Learning & Development Professional of the Year award in her state.

As co-founder of "WTF! Walk the floors," a podcast focused on hospitality training, with a hint of wit she sheds light over the areas of opportunity leaders miss when managing from behind their desk. The podcast turned into a successful training program. As a result, she was recognized within the Top 15 Hospitality Trainers globally.

As a Certified Coach, Michèle also works with individuals 1:1 and in group settings. In 2022 she was selected as one of the Top 5 Coaches to look out for.

As part of her commitment to advocating for DEI&B, she co-founded "We THRIVE," a networking circle aimed to connect, empower, and transform Women.

I HEAR BIRDS CHIRPING

By Michele Kline

For the very first time in about three years, I could hear birds chirping.

I sat down, closed my eyes, and took a deep breath until my lungs were completely full of fresh air. I remember it as if it was yesterday. The beautiful spring morning sun covered my face. It felt warm and particularly bright. I noticed a big pear tree in the corner, blooming at its fullest capacity, gifting us humans with the sweet perfume of its white flowers.

A realization hit me like a six-ton elephant protecting her calf— I had an epiphany.

I could hear birds chirping and the sun on my face!

As hard as I tried, I was unable to remember when the last time I had felt nature with **all** my senses had been.

I have a ritual. Every time I have an epiphany (which I often do) I call my best friend and with the innate enthusiasm that characterizes me, tell her all about it. This time, it was different. This time, I was really scared. I needed time to process it.

The burnout factor felt very real!

According to the dictionary, "burnout" is the reduction of a fuel or substance **to nothing** through combustion. And that, my friend, was exactly what had happened to me. I had none left, zero, rien, nada!

At the time, my career was sucking the life out of me, literally. That day, I became exceedingly aware that I was fully responsible for allowing it to get to that point. It consumed my ability to feel.

As I became aware, I started thinking of the times I found myself staring at my oldest son while he would tell me stories and the information would wash away. I often found myself smiling and nodding, or flat-out asking: "Can you tell me that one more time?" I realized I had not been present for my husband or my parents, and the scariest part of it all was that I had not been nourishing my body and my soul.

It was at this abrupt moment that I was able to register that my life revolved around clients, deadlines, benchmarks, revenue growth, profit margins, key performance indicators, guest satisfaction, and employee retention.

I had forgotten what it felt like to be happy, to enjoy the little things in life like feeling the sun on my face, going for a run, or even literally stopping to smell the roses.

If you have read any of my stories so far, you know by now that I am a humble ninja warrior of my own life. I take responsibility for my behavior. I deeply believe that we are all leaders in this world (in one way or another), and that **leading is a choice.** The way we lead others, but most importantly ourselves, is critical if we want to leave a heroic larger-than-life legacy.

Now, my dear, is when you and I slide together down the rainbow into my little toolbox of life experiences and dig for those tools that make a difference. Ready?

Let's do this!

⚔ **Know your value.** When you are fully aware of the value you bring to your organization, those around you and your own life, you develop a deeper understanding of what you are worth. And trust me, you are worth it!

⚔ **Time is gold.** It is perfectly okay to be jealous with your time. So, make time for yourself. The moment you start owning YOUR time, you start paying attention to what makes you a better human. In the end, we were all placed on this planet to serve, to impact, and to be inspiring.

✖ **Rest.** Resting is absolutely underrated. Make time for it, now. We live in a society that is driven by achievement, qualifications, status, and success. We work arduously to get there day in and day out, and we constantly forget about what our mind and body are telling us. We forget to listen and pay attention to the signs. Now my question is, what is the point of success when we are continuously stressed, tired, and overwhelmed? Do not wait another day. In the end, another day is not guaranteed.

✖ **Say no.** Saying "no" to things you don't want to do is liberating. It's a feeling it took me nearly forty years to acquire. Learn the best way to communicate your needs and wants so that you avoid hurting others with your choices. Start by asking yourself what you *want* to do, instead of what you *should* do. Now, if you want to take it a step further, ask yourself, what is stopping you from saying "no?" "No" is a very powerful word that gives a definitive sense of self. Stop people pleasing because it is not taking you anywhere. Learning to say "no" is the best way to rediscover your priorities and a true sense of who you are.

✖ **Help. Delegate. Empower.** Asking for help and delegating tasks is empowering to those around you. Do more of it! They will appreciate it; you will appreciate it. Delegating and empowering others to get things done helps them build their capabilities and skills. This, in turn, encourages and fosters individual success. Empowered delegation has an array of massive benefits we often are unable to see. Empowerment through delegation will build trust equally in you as it will in others. It also allows those you lead to take on more responsibility. So, do more of it!

🛠 **Authenticity.** Stay authentic to who you are. Your authentic self is who you genuinely are as a human, regardless of your career and the influence of those around you. It is a straightforward representation of you. To be authentic means not paying too much attention to what others think about you. BE you. DO you. All day and every day. This is the secret sauce to allowing yourself to set the right boundaries.

🛠 **Speak up.** Showing that you care and speaking up when something bothers you is crucial for the development of those you care for and those you lead. Most importantly, it is critical to your sanity. Speaking up is an essential part of being honest with others, as well as with yourself. It is honesty that builds trust. More specifically, when combined with tact, the right delivery, and empathy. Never, ever allow anyone to alter your moral compass. BE THE COMPASS.

🛠 **Stop "fixing" people.** Instead, practice giving people the space and time to face the consequences of their behaviors. Stop constantly making a farfetched effort to change or rescue them. Life is all about the choices we make. Everyone makes their bed and should have the courage to sleep in it.

🛠 **Knowing it all.** It is okay to not know everything. Admitting you don't know something, and that you may not have all the answers is completely acceptable. When you find yourself in a situation where you do not have the answer, reach out to others in your network, lean in, and learn to accept. On that same token, avoid getting caught in the whirlwind of having to research for the correct answer, come up with the solution, and resolve everyone's life. Most of the time, what those around you truly need is to feel empowered to go through the process of seeking the answer their own way. Instead, try inspiring them to do so. Be there for them on the sideline.

🛠 **Listen with intent.** Listening without the daunting and heavy feeling of providing solutions is not always needed. You put yourself in this position. I attribute this learning experience solely to my best friend. One day, in a painful tone, she asked me to just listen. She wasn't seeking an answer, she just needed me to listen. She simply needed to vent. Listen with the intent to understand, show sympathy, and be empathetic.

"Stopping to smell the roses," allowing yourself to become aware and listen to the birds chirping is an act of appreciation. Being able to be grateful for everything that we are, is the best way to recognize the grander source of all the good and epic things that fill our lives. It is incredibly vital to make the time to recognize those little, sometimes "insignificant" moments that bring us joy and truly feel what causes that emotion.

The moral of the story is that we are solely responsible for the way we feel, or better yet, for the way we don't feel. We are responsible for our health, our nutrition, and our good and bad habits getting in the way. It is solely up to us to know when to stop, to set boundaries, and allow ourselves to hear the birds chirping!

From that day forward, my key performance indicators (also known as K.P.I.) have shifted. I now keep people interested, keep people informed, keep people involved, keep people in mind, and keep people inspired.

Take control, take action, and take ownership.

Yours truly,
A humble Ninja Warrior of her own life.

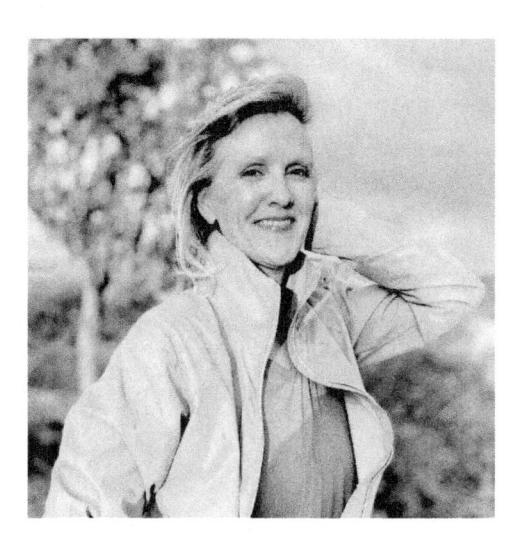

Rebecca Chandler

CEO & Owner of Wholistic Arizona Healing Ranch, Wholistic Finance

https://www.linkedin.com/in/rebecca-chandler-80207b229/
https://www.facebook.com/rebecca.chandler.585
https://twitter.com/wholisticaz
https://wholisticarizona.com/
https://www.wholisticarizona.com/wholisticfinance

A survivor of infant and teenage physical and sexual abuse, Rebecca spent decades confounded with chronic illness, pain, clinical depression, severe anxiety, and panic disorder. She was repeatedly psychoanalyzed and allopathically evaluated as a surgical and pharmaceutical patient. Instead, Rebecca chose to take the long-term healing route to natural, holistic, heart-reviving recovery where she met her Licensed Acupuncturist husband Ron at 35 years old. With his medical help and guidance, Rebecca was able to have her first child at 40, after multiple lost pregnancies in her 20s and 30s. Ron and Rebecca now run Wholistic Arizona Healing Ranch outside Tucson, Arizona where they offer full-service complementary and alternative medicine therapies, as well as community gardening and animal therapy, for individuals and families. Rebecca owns and works with Wholistic Finance as well, which supports Wholistic Arizona in offering discounted and free health-care services for foster and adoptive families in their region.

MOVING THE MOUNTAINS IN YOUR HEART

By Rebecca Chandler

"Ha" is the sound of the Heart in eastern medicine. The Heart is one of the five energetic organ systems of the body. The Heart system is the benevolent ruler or Emperor of the body. It governs the mind including one's ability to think clearly, sleep soundly and talk fluently, and includes the organs of the heart and small intestine. Within Traditional Chinese Medicine (TCM), the Heart is the most important organ system. It is protected by all other systems and bodily functions.

When one's Heart system is strong and balanced, one's eyes will sparkle with luster and spirit, and one's Heart vitality will manifest in clarity of speech, gentleness of reactions, and brightness of overall appearance. If you ever become hindered by stuttering or insomnia, you are experiencing Heart out of balance. Seeing someone with a red, purple or pale face can also be signals that their Heart is out of balance. The heart organ may be fine and healthy, but the energy of the Heart system may be blocked or otherwise disrupted.

I have been told that the gift of my heart will be a light to others. For much of my life, I have slept poorly, been burdened by over-rumination, felt overwhelmed often, had darkening color to my eyes and skin, and had an emergency-like hyper-reactivity to pretty much all stimuli. It was hard to imagine that a heart with so much stress could be a blessing to others.

My husband and I have been running a natural medicine clinic on our 7-acre ranch outside Tucson, AZ, for 13 years now. He is a licensed Acupuncturist and Traditional Medicine herbalist, in practice since 1985. Both of us have been patients of his care protocols. Our ranch is a retreat for ourselves and our patients. Here, we have developed many healing practices to balance our Hearts and to bring overall health and peace to our bodies and lives.

Through our healing work, I now sleep better, have clarity of thought, less anxiety, and my skin and eyes are much brighter – even to the point when meeting strangers, they sometimes blurt out: "well, you're a bright light!" It is due to the marvelous healing power of our Wholistic 5-part healing system which transcends physical health, allowing both broken Hearts *and* ill bodies such as mine the opportunity to mend.

In over 70 years of combined healing experiences, my husband and I have witnessed amazing longevity improvements and health, and have condensed them into 5 Healing Steps with which we coach our clients:

1. Purify your blood
2. Nourish your cells
3. Strengthen & balance your energy
4. Nurture your spirit
5. Serve & lift others

Our Hearts act as controller to the fountain of our blood. Our minds think clearly when our blood is clean. In order to purify our blood, our first Healing Step is colon hydrotherapy and herbal detoxification. This Step allows the body to purge environmental and dietary toxins from our cells that can cause pallor of skin, liver spots, cloudy thinking and other distresses to mind and body. Step 1 had the immediate result of reducing my headaches, and lightening the age and liver spotting on the sides of my face and neck that had been slowly creeping up for decades.

Our second Healing Step is to nourish our cells by consuming a primarily organic, raw, free-range, as-local-as-possible diet of grains, vegetables, and fruits in season, plus raw dairy and supplemental organic free-range meats. Our bodies obtain nutrients needed to sustain life from the food we eat, so our body can be fully nourished when our food is fresh and rich in energy and nutrition. We cut out packaged foods wherever possible and teach our clients how to make homemade versions of most everything we consume.

Alongside these, we begin Step 3, using acupuncture, moxibustion and traditional herbal therapies to repair and remove old trauma and blocked energy in the Heart and body. Acupuncture and TCM herbs promote, restore, and maintain health by bringing balance and order to the energy of the body. Pain and emotional distress will block and disrupt the Heart and other systems causing short and long-term illness. Shocking experiences in infancy and youth had marred much of my Heart energy, which was underlying the many imbalances in my health. I have been practicing these first 3 Steps for over 18 years and have made super strides towards balancing my Heart to move the old damage out, making space for the gift and light to come.

Cleaning out the old toxins, replenishing with pure foods, and strengthening our nervous systems are the physical foundations of health we have discovered. But more than physical health is required to enjoy full wellness and truly move the mountains in your Heart. We joined our church in 2014. As we began to treat church members in our clinic practice, we noticed one amazing thing: they had a baseline of health we had never seen before, even without cellular cleansing, eating pure foods, and receiving strengthening treatments. We were floored! But it made sense as we pondered on it. One of the central tenets of our faith is that we are beloved children of our Heavenly Father, and one of the central practices of our faith is to receive the gift of the Holy Spirit. Our church members feel LOVED and filled with heavenly inspiration! This love and inspiration bring a higher level of basic health than we had witnessed in over 35 years of professional practice. We became true believers that nurturing our spirit and feeling loved were paramount in finding true, lasting health and wellness.

Our last step to whole health is to serve and lift others. Reviews of prison and hostage camp accounts reveal that those who survived best were those who were concerned for their fellow prisoners, and who were willing to give away their own food and substance to help sustain others. And in a 5,000 member survey conducted by United Healthcare and Volunteer Match, they found that the act of serving others, in itself, can increase one's level of happiness, yielding a sense of purpose and an increased amount of self-esteem. When these qualities are present, in the TCM paradigm, all body energies will be flowing at optimal rates, providing highest conditions for best overall health!

My journey in life commenced with 20 years of intermittent abuse. While the abuses were hidden by nighttime and drugging, my subconscious and cellular memory were heavily burdened. I have completed 18 years of the first 3 steps and 8 years of all 5 steps. In those last 8 years of the 5 steps combined, I have found exponential relief of the physical and emotional poisons embedded in my body and soul.

This kind of relief from and release of trauma and toxicity bring the best opportunity for overall health and wellness. As the body is cleansed, strengthened, and nourished, there will be more energy flowing to the Heart. As the Heart is nurtured, supported, comforted, and filled, the body will swell with supernatural ability to heal and be well. Hope will abound and joy will be felt freely.

Other than persons born with birth defects, each soul on earth is born with a strong heart and strong mind. Mothering, natural birth, bonding and loving care each support the energy of the Heart, filling it with sufficient strength to carry it through a lifetime of work, play and myriad experiences. Lacking self-love, having fear and judgment, or lacking the feeling of being loved will all deplete the energy of the Heart. When you have clean blood and have released trauma from your cells, you are more open to feeling loved by our Heavenly source, our father in Heaven and His son Jesus Christ.

I still fall back into chest-shaking heart-pounding malaise sometimes. This happens when I am letting go of deep-rooted shock or trauma. But I can feel joy as those experiences are released. When I start having headaches again or become irritable, my daughter will remind me it is time for Step 1 again. Daily, we as a family practice Steps 2, 4 & 5. Step 3 is a gift for us when we can get on my husband's clinic schedule. He has even taught our 12-year-old daughter to effectively insert his acupuncture needles so that as a healer, he may be healed too.

With all the tools available to each of us now, we have everything needed to heal from the poison lifestyle in our world, the toxic relationships of society and the lack of faith in humanity. All the necessary tools for true health and wellness are here. As we use the earthly and heavenly tools in our 5 Healing Steps, and coach our clients through them, we see mountains of old emotional garbage released and disposed; we see mountains of pain and hardship removed; we see mountains of hurt healed in the hearts of family and friends.

Rebecca Chandler, Owner Wholistic Arizona Healing Ranch

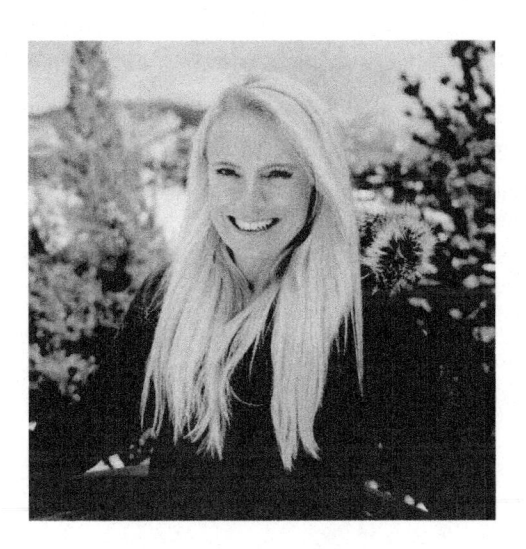

Amanda O'Mara

Founder & CEO of Impact Coach Mastermind and Lift Like a Boss Fitness Business Coach

www.instagram.com/amanda_omara_/
www.facebook.com/amanda.omara/
www.linkedin.com/in/amanda-o-mara-7a5730177/
www.amandaomara.com
www.amandaomara.com/impactcoachmastermindphoenix

Amanda O'Mara is an unstoppable woman with a passionate power to help others step into their true potential as an online fitness entrepreneur, knowing this will create a ripple effect in the health and wellness industry worldwide. She is on a mission to impact millions by transforming their lives and their bank accounts.

She was born in Michigan, raised in New Hampshire and is now settled in the mountains of Colorado in a home that she and her husband built after losing everything to a wildfire.

She is a fitness business coach, certified personal trainer and nutritionist, writer, life coach, speaker and dog mom. Amanda also got her B.A. in Hospitality at Metropolitan State University of Denver then worked her way in restaurants for nearly a decade. After learning what good service really means, thousands now come to her for her expertise and support in building an online fitness business.

BEAUTY FROM ASHES: A HEALING PATH FOR THE MIND, BODY & SOUL

By Amanda O'Mara

In my experience, victims ask, "Why me?" and survivors ask, "What now?" I've been both.

It was the evening of October 21st, 2020 when my dog and I left in terror and made a run for our lives.

Rewind a couple of years. I had built a multi six-figure online health and fitness business, triumphed through trauma therapy, bought our forever dream home in the mountains, and was in the best shape of my life—both in mind and body.

But in the blink of an eye, my life forever changed.

It was one of the most rapid-fire expansions ever, and Colorado's second-largest wildfire in record history. With no evacuation order, I was home when the air turned deep red all around me.

I was standing in the kitchen of our recently bought home when I saw our neighbor's house on fire and a wave of flames coming rapidly towards me.

As I was dropping the f-bomb, I grabbed my dog and ran out of the house as quickly as I could. It came so fast the lights were left on, the front door wide open, and packed bags were left piled up in the mudroom.

Smoke and fire now surrounded the premises.

I was on the phone with my husband, Mike, a firefighter, screaming in disbelief. With a trailer attached to my Jeep, I slammed on the gas and made my way down the hill. Within thirty seconds, I lost connection on the phone with him—for about twenty minutes I had no service.

The heat and winds were so bad, and trees were falling and being uplifted by the roots and slamming into the trailer and my car as I was escaping. One fell on the front bumper and rammed up through the radiator and into the engine.

The car kept going for about four more miles before it broke down.

As I stepped out of the car to call for help, it was pure chaos. The town had started to evacuate. Both lanes were open as there was only one road out.

Soon, my husband found me and we got the heck out of there.

Within 24 hours, the fire went from 18,550 acres to 187,964 acres, killing two people, many animals, and destroying over 400 homes and structures. Our home was one of them.

It happened during Covid, when building costs skyrocketed overnight and everyone was underinsured.

I endured severe PTSD, anxiety, and depression for months to follow. My hair started thinning and acne surfaced as stress was at an all-time high. I struggled to breathe for a while because my lungs were damaged by the smoke.

My coaching business took a turn for the worse as well.

I paid the last of what I had left in my bank account to my team to finish what was needed for our clients. I thought, "How can I coach someone to take care of their health and coach business when I am mentally gone?"

Shortly after, the business shut down for many months.

Have you ever been so deeply hurt that not even a whole bottle of whiskey can make you feel drunk? Stress and pain can do that sometimes. It feels extremely lonely and you may lose interest in the things you once loved. You may feel low in energy or be overly tired. You may even begin to feel guilty for what you did or didn't do. You can lose a sense of hope, a sense of self and wonder if it will ever end.

Your body is stuck in constant fight or flight response. Your body feels like it wants to shut down, and your mental health could lead to feeling like giving up on everything, including life. I get it, because that was me too.

But through the kindness of people, my therapist, energy healers, and an introduction to plant medicine—I was slowly able to find myself again and you can too.

Many have asked me, "How did you start improving your health again to get out of a deep and dark funk?" It wasn't going to the gym again or just eating chicken and broccoli. That felt overwhelming and intimidating. (By the way, this is a normal feeling when starting anything new or getting back into a routine.) Instead, I started with a very simple step that anyone can do no matter how stuck you feel. Begin with gratitude.

Getting into the energy of gratitude, will create a ripple effect in helping you create healthier habits. From gratitude, taking the next step will be easier. Think of very small changes you can make just today, like choosing an apple instead of a bag of chips or sitting down for three minutes to journal.

Only look back to see how far you've come. I was reminded by my past clients why I was here, and I started receiving daily messages like:

"Coach, I just hit my first $10,000 month!"

"Hey Coach, I can't thank you enough… I just signed on five more clients this month!"

"Amanda, thank you for your help… I wanted to let you know that I just lost 21 pounds and started therapy."

As I grew stronger mentally, my body did too.

I started to lift weights again, drank less alcohol, and absorbed as many nutritious foods as I could.

With patience, consistency, and trust in myself, I was reborn. I became stronger and healthier and found a 'no-BS' confidence I never knew I had. Confidence of self-belief, self-love, and less worry about what other people thought of me.

Within a few months, I re-launched my business and hit a record-breaking month. Today, I have a team of five incredible humans sharing a similar mission to impact the health and fitness space by the masses.

We won't stop until our deathbed to transform minds, bodies, and bank accounts one at a time.

So why do I share my story with you? Suffering is universal. We will be affected by environmental and genetic factors over which we have little or no control.

We sometimes ask "Why did this happen to me?" and think this could lessen the pain. Why did he sexually abuse me? Why did my parents abandon me? Why do I have cancer? Why did I lose my job? Why am I so broke all the time?

As humans, we search for logic and answers but when we ask why, we end up staying stuck searching for blame—including ourselves. But we each get to choose whether or not we stay a victim. We don't get to choose what happens to us, but we do get to choose how we respond to our experiences.

So, my advice to you when all feels lost, is to move forward with a gentle embrace and start with gratitude. Learn what you need in the present moment and take your next step from there. Take radical responsibility even in situations you did not choose. Freedom comes with a price and a willingness to let go and grow.

I'd also like to note that trauma is relative. My story may come off as extreme to some, but to me, it's nothing compared to the many lives and homes lost in Ukraine.

Trauma is any event that disrupts our emotional functioning. It should not be labeled as "Big-T" or "Little-T." Trauma is trauma. It all matters, and it impacts each person differently.

Trauma can surface in many shapes and forms in our bodies. For me, it was panic attacks, depression, and digestive issues. For others, it could be anxiety, OCD, cancer, and thyroid problems.

In a way, it is our body's way of screaming for help.

Listen to it, pay attention to it, and take care of it like you would a child. You too were once a child and that inner-child is still within us. If your inner-child asked you to take care of her right now, what would you do for her? What would you say to her? What would tell her to believe? How would you nurture her? Love her unconditionally, give her patience and grace, and trust her potential to do what she's always wanted to do. Believe in her.

Move your body in a way that feels best to you. Lift weights in the gym, do some Yoga, go hiking, try boxing, train for a mud race, stretch, go mountain biking, or simply just walk the dog or get off the couch. Just move and get the blood flowing.

Fuel your body with nutritious foods. Prioritize protein in every meal, eat different colors of the rainbow every day with fruits and vegetables, and please just eat the damn carbs. Carbs are our main source of energy, and we need them to function optimally. Drink a gallon of water a day. Above all, eat consciously and enjoy each bite like it's your last.

Take care of your soul and your energy. Protect it with healthy boundaries. Find ways to connect and be calm. Meditate for ten minutes a day, name three things you're grateful for when you wake up, journal out intentions and affirmations, be in nature, visualize for thirty seconds about your goals in life, or take a hot bath with Epsom salt and candlelight.

Flex your brain muscles. Did you know that if you train your brain properly, you can improve the connective tissues between the neurons in your brain to help them work better and faster? You can improve cognition by simply reading a book, trying a new sport, cooking a new dish, or investing in a course to gain more knowledge in a specialty you've always wanted to try.

As a reminder, when life interrupts us or stops us in our tracks there is always a transition. Let it be a catalyst to emerge from victimhood and decide what is next for you. Whether you're working on your health journey or starting a business, keep going.

XO
Amanda O'Mara

P.s. If you are in the health space and are looking to start an online business, I have some juicy nuggets for you to take away today. Here is a step-by-step blueprint to help get you started so you know exactly how to build a $10k+ month online business that you love.

#1.) Niche down. Know what target market and main problem you want to solve. Doing this will allow you to stand out, charge high prices, attract dream clients, and create better content.

#2.) Create a high ticket offer, because those who pay, pay attention. And those who pay attention, get better results. Win, win! Oh, and because you're worth it!

#3.) First master a daily client attraction system organically through social media. Why not, it's free! Plus, it will give you a chance to dial in your marketing message to attract leads who are ready to pay you large sums of money before you blindly throw it at paid advertising.

#4.) Make sales sexy. Sales shouldn't be salesy, pushy, or weird. Learn the skills behind it and avoid cold direct selling. Know it's a service. You have a gift, share it. Besides, you just can't have a business without sales.

#5.) Great coaching begins with a smooth client onboarding process, asking them the right questions, daily/weekly check-ins, and offboarding processes. Client fulfillment is key to client retention and growth.

#6:) The most important, yet the most overlooked piece, is the consistent work on bringing out your CEO mindset, even if you think you have a good head on your shoulders. Success will come from 80% mindset and 20% systems and strategies. If you don't believe in yourself, why should your clients?

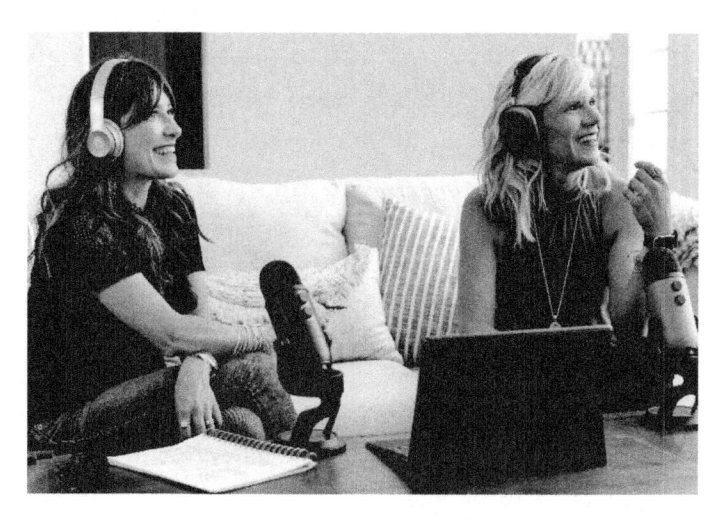

Natasha Ganes and Jennifer Griffith

Founders of In the Life of Zen

https://www.instagram.com/inthelifeofzen/
https://www.facebook.com/inthelifeofzen
https://www.linkedin.com/company/inthelifeofzen/
https://inthelifeofzen.com/

Jen and Natasha have been friends and occasional co-conspirators for many years, but it wasn't until 2019 that they decided to join forces and combine their areas of expertise, which includes over 35 years of combined experience in health, wellness, and professional development.

They created In the Life of Zen and the Where Money Meets Soul podcast as a way to share those tools and resources with others, so that they too can turn their desires into reality.

Stress management, success, financial freedom, work/life balance, abundance – whatever you want to create in your life, you can have it and they can help you get there. Sometimes all it takes to achieve your goals is a tribe of people cheering you on and wanting you to succeed and they're here to do just that for each one of you.

PRIORITIZE SELF-CARE TO AVOID BURNOUT

By Natasha Ganes and Jennifer Griffith

We all feel the effects of stress at some time or another, and while feeling it every now and again is fine (in fact some stress is beneficial), an abundance of it can cause our minds and bodies to overreact, make us sick, and lead to burnout. To avoid that, you must prioritize your self-care, which can feel difficult to do. The good news is that there are many ways to do that and all of them can be incorporated into your daily routine. The key is to find the ways that resonate and work for you.

When you prioritize self-care, your mind, body, and soul reap the benefits, which allows you to become the best version of yourself and helps you live your best life.

Natasha's Story

Everyone wants to live their best life. Sometimes though, we're not sure what that looks like. We know we have talents or things we like to do, but we don't know how to incorporate them into our lives. Maybe we want to save money, start a new business, change careers, or simply live a more fulfilled life, but we worry we won't succeed. We know there is more we could do, but we aren't quite sure what that is. Trust me, I get it.

As a busy woman who always has a lot of balls in the air, I know what it's like to live with stress and overwhelm. At one point in my career, I could not get a handle on my stress—it consumed my entire life and left me overwhelmed.

Jennifer's Story

I'm one of those people who always needs to be doing something. I need to feel productive, constantly checking things off both the real and proverbial lists and getting stuff done. From the moment I wake up to the moment I fall asleep, I am usually on the go.

I have also worked from home since 2008 and have a corporate job that demands a lot of my attention. For years, my morning commute consisted of exiting my bedroom, entering the kitchen to grab a cup of coffee and breakfast, and walking into my office to begin my day. From about 10 minutes after I woke up until the moment I went to bed, my mind was constantly working and ON. I worked this way for years until I slowly started to feel like I was sacrificing myself for the demands of my job, home, family, bills, etc. This is when I completely burnt out. I was too exhausted to want to do anything and slowly found myself in a funk. I lead myself to an unhappy place before I questioned: *How did I get here? Why did I let this happen?*

Overwhelm, Stress & Burn Out

It's easy to feel stressed out and overwhelmed. It's also easy to go on for years living in a dominant state of overwhelm without giving it much thought until something occurs that forces us to realize we've been on autopilot. Overwhelm can get you so caught up in your thoughts and emotions that you lack efficacy in your life. After time, it leads to higher stress and anxiety levels and strips you of overall joy and satisfaction.

Many things can lead to overwhelm and a perfect 50/50 work/life balance does not exist. However, putting your needs first with self-care is an absolute must to avoid burnout. Signs of burnout can include a combination of the following:

- Exhaustion over even the smallest tasks
- Irritation at home and work
- Forgetfulness
- Lack of energy/motivation/satisfaction/concentration
- Procrastination
- Compulsive worrying

- Negative emotions
- Change in sleeping habits
- Unexplained health issues, such as headaches, stomachaches, etc.

We both know what it's like to feel stressed out, overwhelmed, and burnt out. We also know how to pull ourselves out of that place by using the right skills and tools to get our lives into alignment.

Studies prove that when you prioritize your spiritual, physical, and mental health, it leads to a more balanced, happier life. Your overall health affects how you think, feel, and act. Self-care plays a significant role in maintaining your health and helps support treatment and recovery when you are not doing well.

Prioritizing self-care is vital to your overall wellbeing.

When we refer to self-care, we mean creating a daily, sustainable practice that keeps you mentally and physically healthy. Even the smallest bit of daily self-care can make an enormous difference in your life. It helps you manage stress, increases your energy, and lowers your risk of illness. However, it can be difficult to maintain a healthy work/life balance when you're juggling everything that life throws your way. Some people even find it easier to stay busy instead of relaxing, which keeps them in a state of high-functioning anxiety. In your rush to get everything done, you forget that when your stress levels rise, your productivity and concentration drop, which makes you feel irritable and anxious and takes a toll on your happiness and wellbeing.

While a certain amount of stress is beneficial and can help you perform at your best; prolonged stress and the lack of a healthy work/life balance has detrimental consequences. Unfortunately, if you do not take care of yourself first your health will suffer, and you will end up living in the land of overwhelm and burnout. To avoid that, you must prioritize self-care and create healthy boundaries. Here are a few ideas to help:

Write Down Everything You Need to Do and Learn to Delegate

Instead of struggling to remember all the things you need to do, write them down in order of importance. If something doesn't have to get done right now, remove it from the list and save it for another day, or delegate it to someone else.

Accept Your Emotions and Change Your Perspective

What you focus on grows, so instead of thinking about everything you have to do, accept how you feel and then take a break to count your blessings and send some gratitude out into the universe. It may sound silly or trite, but training your mind to flip the switch from panic to appreciation in moments of high stress can often mean the difference between a life of anxiety and one of peace.

Create Boundaries and Stick with Them

You don't need to agree to everything that's thrown your way. If it's a friend who is asking for your time, explain that you can't fit it into your schedule, but you appreciate the offer. If it's your boss or a client, tell them that given your workload, the task would be difficult for you to complete at this time, but perhaps there is another way to get it done. The more you practice saying no, the easier it will become.

Exercise

Start by incorporating 30 minutes of exercise each day. If you don't have a full 30 minutes, take two 15-minute breaks or three 10-minute breaks. Exercise will not only help to enrich your quality of life, but it leads to a more positive attitude as well.

Practice Mindfulness

An easy way to do this is to sit silently, take slow and deep breaths for

2-3 minutes, and focus your thoughts on each breath.

Try Something New

Do an activity that's out of the ordinary for you, such as test driving a sports car, going to the movies by yourself, learning how to knit, sky diving, reading a classic novel, or taking a surf lesson or a salsa dancing class. Anything that makes you feel proud of yourself for taking a risk.

Take a Digital Detox

Once a day for at least one hour, turn off all your devices. Use the time that you would usually spend staring at a screen on self-care activities, like meditating, hiking, or taking a nap or bath.

Meditate

If you don't already meditate or believe you don't know how to meditate, guided meditations are a great way to start. Research shows that just five minutes a day helps to reduce stress and control anxiety.

Sleep

Each night start by relaxing about 90 minutes before going to bed: diffuse lavender oil; take a hot shower or bath to relax muscles, lower body tension, and reduce anxiety; or sit in silence and turn off all electronics to avoid overstimulating your brain.

The goal is to get to a point where prioritizing self-care is a non-negotiable part of your life. Self-care is a form of self-preservation that optimizes your mental, physical, and spiritual health. Do this and you will become unstoppable!

If it weren't for these powerful tools, we wouldn't be where we are today. *In the Life of Zen* shares our experiences and lessons, so that you can use that knowledge to help you create the life of your dreams.

Jennifer & Natasha

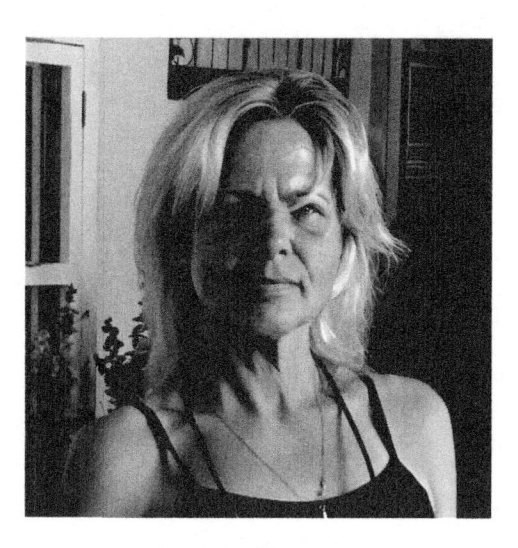

Andra Annette

Pounds-to-Go
Nurse/Holistic Practitioner

https://www.facebook.com/andra.annette
https://www.instagram.com/coachpro50/
https://www.linkedin.com/in/andra-annette-621a21101/
https://pounds-to-go.com
https://heal.me/andraannette

Worked in Health care 35 years. Private Practice Nutritionist at Pounds-to go. Overcoming my own weight loss struggles, thyroid condition, and auto-immune disorders, I now work with other women to help them achieve weight loss. By developing a new relationship with food, they learn to use nutrition to support their bodies and live in a body they love. My journey as a health coach started in 2020 while being a nurse on the front lines. I saw the impact lifestyle choices had on outcomes and knew I could help more women with strategies and nutritional concepts that lead to optimal health.

HOPE'S PROMISE

By Andra Annette

When hope feels distant, I close my eyes and the smell of sweet hydrangeas fills me, soothing me even now. Funny how fond memories of our formative years can still fill us with warmth like no other known. Mary Marrow was my nanny as a child and my earliest memory of peace. Her yard was my amusement park. Big blooming hydrangea trees in a variety of colors flooded the yard. Through the back gate, a small store owner sold penny candies I would delight in often. My sisters were coming to take me home soon.

The years progressed. Sure, a house of five girls would have their disagreements, but it was us against the world. Many people have doctors, teachers, and accountants that they may also aspire to be when they grow up. My mom had no formal education and no high school diploma until much later in her life. I may not have had something to aspire to, but I had a strong support system. A family who loved and believed in me.

Self-Concept

Perception is a powerful motivator, yet it can also be a source of discontent. What does it matter if someone loves you if at your core you feel unworthy? I always thought I was adopted. My sister Laura was mean-spirited by nature and would tell us that growing up. Laura would go on to say that, if I did not behave, I would be shipped back to where I came from. The thought would resonate and remain somewhere in my mind. Always feeling like I didn't belong anywhere.

I would spend a great deal of my life people-pleasing and trying to fit in, becoming lost to my true self. From the exterior, I appeared happy, but underneath I struggled. The only time I would express myself was in my writing. Did you ever feel polite indifference? Living a life of muddling through always yearning for more?

As children, you're reminded to be grateful for all that you have, implying that you're ungrateful if you want more, often taught you must work hard to succeed. I would spend decades straying away from things that were easy because I believed they had no value. There was a deep seeded root that left a fear. Afraid of failing at what I truly loved, I would decide not to explore those options. Another part of my alter ego was afraid of succeeding. The one time I remember being happy was fleeting and accompanied by a tragedy.

I admired people who smiled all the time and truly looked happy. People confused me, which started my fascination with watching and listening earnestly. I would sit at my window as a young woman and watch them for long periods, curious to know their secret.

I would have extreme highs and extreme lows growing up and was prone to hormonal disorders. There were few I shared my true emotions with and now understand I suffered from depression. I attributed my feelings to peer pressure. All those feelings would lie bottled inside and keep me emotionally stuck as a child.

I allowed people to treat me in ways less than I deserved. I spent years in an abusive marriage believing that was all I deserved. One day, finally ready to say goodbye to that daily life, I would hear my mother in my head saying, "There are no victims, just volunteers. "People only treat you the way you allow them to." I would end that marriage. All those years of holding in all that pain would surface and become a strength now that I needed it. I regained that inner child I left alone for so long.

I spent the next year alone. For the first time ever I wasn't someone's girlfriend, friend, sister, daughter, or wife. Learning to say no became freeing. I did things just for enjoyment's sake. I no longer cared what anyone thought I should or shouldn't do for a living or with my life.

Signs

As early as six I knew I wanted to work with people. People-watching was my favorite pastime. Well, that and science. Little did I know that I would find a way to combine them. I would head to college and pursue my childhood dream of helping others as a nurse. I can still see my mom's face beaming with pride at my graduation.

My career would take me on many different paths as I learned different facets of nursing and settled into different roles. The role that most appealed to me over my career was geriatrics. I lived in an elderly community at the time that embraced me and I them.

I always felt they were the forgotten ones. Family members who could not manage their family members' advancing disease processes would leave them in our care. Some returned to visit, but many would not. They would become my family away from home.

Out of Self into Others.

Nursing can be a stressful job. Usually, I thrived in that environment, but one day that changed. Healthcare became more about business than about the people it served. More tasks were added, staffing cut, and it was harder to give people the quality care they needed and deserved. I stayed daily without pay to ensure they received what they needed. I worked in several managerial roles in nursing, but I always ended up at the bedside.

My oldest sister, Dee, would die suddenly at 49 years old and my mother shortly thereafter. Horrified at the caregivers they sent to help my mom, my sister, Denise, and I alternated that role as needed. I requested time off and would be told it wasn't a good time. I got a call from Denise that mom was rushed to the hospital, and I left that day and never returned.

My sister Denise and I remained with mom until her imminent death. The impact of mom's death was too much to endure. I still hadn't grieved my oldest sister fully, and I became overwhelmed with a sense of hopelessness. Now losing two of the three most important women in my life brought me to my knees. Knowing I could not care for others in this state of emotional turmoil, I took the next year away from nursing.

I withdrew from others to reevaluate life on life's terms. I returned after taking a year off to work on my own health. The stress of the last few years had brought all my autoimmune diseases out in force. Never being formally diagnosed until years later I again treated myself for the problems I knew always existed. I started my nursing career at 110 pounds and here I stood at 257 pounds hating the girl in the mirror. Depression stopped me from eating but working long hours as a nurse stopped me from eating at any real scheduled times. A real killer of thyroid disease.

I had studied nutrition independently with thyroid and autoimmune diseases. I went back to the treatments I created for myself that I knew worked. As much as we want to believe appearance doesn't matter, it does matter to self-confidence. The real change came when I acknowledged I could and would do this. I knew from experience that restrictive diets didn't work, so I focused on daily habits I could change.

I had before been able to keep my illnesses at bay, but grief changed me. My job and lifestyle were full of stress, which was an autoimmune disease breeding ground. I got back into a semblance of life and focused on putting my diseases at bay again.

I had several disease processes that remained asymptomatic for a decade. I combined nursing science with nutrition to give myself a quality life. We set our own limits in life. Our upbringing or outside influences play a part in that but it's a choice to let those limits define how your life moves forward. Fears can't be what holds us back.

I returned to work, changed focus, and worked for the city in public health. I am part of New York City's emergency response team. Covid happened and I was not sure if we would be sent yet, but knew I was going in even if it was as a volunteer. I remember my husband saying, "You're going in, aren't you?" I am grateful he understood it was something I had to do, and he was confident in my abilities.

We were there for a long time, and I saw things I had never seen before in my nursing career. Despite everything going on around me, I felt a strange piece of me come alive. This was where I belonged helping others. Many lives would be lost during Covid. Parents, husbands, daughters, and good people would never make it home.

They said lifestyle choices were a contributing factor in disease outcomes and so at night after my shifts, I studied and became a holistic practitioner. I wanted to help more and reach people before it was too late. I wanted to focus on prevention and curative holistic medicine rather than symptom management.

Listening Fully

Planning to move away from nursing kept me at odds with myself. Starting your own business is scary at first. Questions like "Can I do this?" What if it doesn't work out? What if it does? Planning to make the biggest impact I chose weight loss for my business. Who knows if the circumstances we go through choose us so that we can share that experience and hope with someone else.

Obesity continues to be on the rise leading to other disease processes. Helping people lose weight is an ideal way to prevent those other diseases and allow them to show up for their families while enjoying their best lives. Health is a gift; one many take for granted until it changes. Living with autoimmune and thyroid disease has given me a clear view and knowledge of how important.

I help women lose weight and keep it off by using my lifestyle blueprint method, not another diet. I was able to lose 100lbs using my methods and stop dieting more than a decade ago. I am a weight loss and hormone expert but specialize in gut health because there is a definitive link to all other health-related diseases. I am an expert in thyroid and autoimmune disease because I live with three of my own.

Society puts so much emphasis on appearance even though it's a very small component of who we are as people. My programs do have modalities in mindset to help improve self-esteem. Stress management is another component because stress is killing achievable outcomes in weight loss. I help people develop a new relationship with food.

I love seeing women get results they never thought possible so they can live in a body they love as the best version of themselves. I see many other aspects of their health improve while working with me.

Many people think of weight loss as physical but there's a big emotional component many do not see. I am alarmed at the number of young people today who suffer from body image disturbance, from the amount of bullying people have been exposed to over appearance in society today. Studies show children start dieting as early as six or seven because they are already experiencing dissatisfaction with their bodies. As a society, we can do better.

I hope someday our journeys will cross. I am now on a mission to empower every living person with the knowledge to heal their minds and body through optimal nutrition, daily movement, and consistent action.

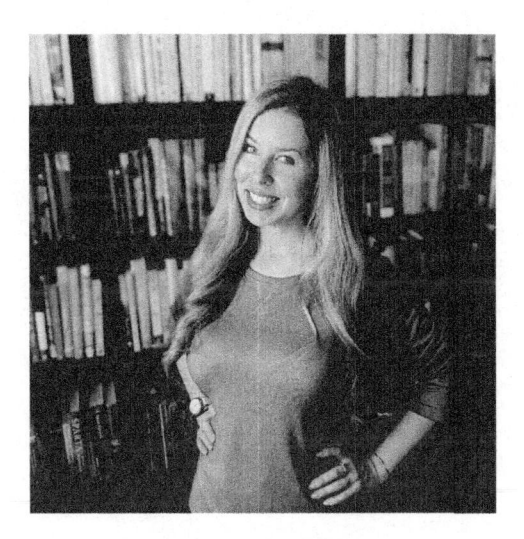

Olivia Radcliffe

Founder/Creator/Co-founder of The Bluebell Group/
The Mom Boss Society/Like a Mother Movement

https://www.linkedin.com/in/momboss-olivia-radcliffe/
www.instagram.com/thebluebellgroup
https://www.facebook.com/thebluebellgroup
www.thebluebellgroup.com
www.likeamothermovement.com

Boy Mom, Dog Mom, Marketing Coach, and Mom Boss Extraordinaire. Olivia Radcliffe is a much sought-after expert in all things marketing. Olivia specializes in helping mompreneurs scale their businesses to 6+ figures without sleazy sales tactics, so they can focus on what really matters most to them. She firmly believes that women don't have to choose between being a great mom/wife/partner and being a successful entrepreneur.

Olivia is also a women empowerment speaker, podcast host, international bestselling author, and co-founder of the like a mother movement. Spending time with family is incredibly important to

Olivia, and when she's not collaborating with other amazing mompreneurs, she can usually be found on a walk with her toddler and german shepherd. To learn more about Olivia and how she can help you grow your business, visit https://thebluebellgroup.com or www.likeamothermovement.com

WITH YOUR NEXT EXHALE...

By Olivia Radcliffe

"Learn how to exhale. The inhale will take care of itself."
—Carla Melucci Ardito

Quick question for you—

When someone asks you how you're doing, how often does your answer involve the word "busy"?

When I first decided to pay attention to this within my own conversations, I was a bit taken aback to realize how often I used the B word.

Oh, you know, I'm just busy! Things are nonstop. How are you?

I wasn't surprised that I was busy—I'm a solo mom with multiple businesses, a household to run, and an almost masochistic need to always have a DIY home project ongoing. I *know* I'm busy.

But, despite my continually full plate, I seldom *feel* busy anymore. So why was I declaring it over and over again?

We are in an epidemic of busyness, where being "busy" is not only the norm, it's almost worn as a badge of honor. If you're not overwhelmed and stressed with everything you're juggling daily, then you are not doing enough.

A lot of the busyness is also self-imposed. A good deal of this histrionic exhaustion we face is an attempt to reassure ourselves that we are useful, we have a purpose, and to mask feelings of not being worthy.

But the biggest irony of all? *We're not even all that busy.*

Hold up—before you throw the book down and get back to cooking dinner while helping your first grader with her homework and pre-treating your son's soccer uniform, let me explain.

We all certainly have a lot to juggle day in and day out, and it no doubt takes its toll on us, but the bigger feelings of stress, exhaustion, and overwhelm come mainly from how we go about these tasks, not from the number of tasks themselves.

When my son was an infant, I would actually get angry when well-meaning people would advise me to sleep while the baby slept. *Of course* I wanted to sleep, I was exhausted to the point of tears. But his naptime was also my only opportunity to pump and sterilize the bottles and feed myself, which were also essential tasks.

And as my son grew, so did my to-do list. As a mompreneur, multitasking wasn't just a talent, it was a survival tactic. And I was *brilliant* at it.

But I noticed that my short-term memory started to lapse. I would forget what I was saying mid-sentence. I was losing track of what day it was. And at the end of the day after I put my son to bed, it was all I could do to curl up in bed myself and fall into a fitful sleep full of dreams of my to-do lists.

It was one night when I woke up and automatically started writing an email in a half-dream state that I decided something had to change.

As my task load couldn't realistically change, I decided to take a deeper look at how I went about my tasks and discovered four key perspective shifts that foundationally changed my life.

The Main Thing is to Keep the Main Thing the Main Thing

I decided to consciously stop multitasking as much. Our brains were designed to focus on one key task at a time. When we multitask and force our brain to jump from one task to another and back again, the brain actually takes *more* time to do tasks, and we end up with memory impairment, problems focusing, and increased stress levels.

While some level of multitasking was inevitable, I started being very intentional with each thing I did, focusing completely on what I was doing in the moment. If I was playing cars with my son, I wasn't also checking my emails on my phone. If I was answering an email, I wasn't also looking at Facebook.

I quickly found that not only did it feel like I was doing less and I was able to get more done, but I also felt better about the *quality* of work I was doing.

Yoga, along with other forms of movement like Tai Chi, incorporates the focus of connecting your breath with your movements. This intentionality helps increase your awareness of both your breath and your body; you'll be more keenly aware of when you are holding your breath, if you are tensing certain muscles, etc.

Having this same intentionality and focus as you work on your tasks throughout the day will help you to be aware of things that might have otherwise gone unnoticed, see details that might have been missed, and feel a sense of joy that might have otherwise been masked by the need to go, go, go.

Appreciate the Baby Steps

My businesses are like my babies. I absolutely love what I do and the women I get to work with, and can honestly say that each day I wake up excited about how we're impacting the world. So it can be frustrating, to say the least, when there are things I know I need to do to help encourage that growth, but I don't have the time nor the mental bandwidth to do them. But the reality is that the destination is pointless without the journey because it is the journey that prepares us for the destination.

If you're ready to fly with something, it can be exasperating to stare up at the sky and feel your feet firmly on the ground. So understand the sky is there—and you will get there—but bring your focus back down to the first small baby step you need to take. Before you know it, your steps will pick up momentum and you'll be running, jumping, and then flying.

The Doing and the Being

When you have a lot to do, it's easy to get swept up in the masculine energy of taking action and the need to DO. Every waking moment (and some non-waking ones) becomes about hustling to *get it all done*.

If you focus all of your energy, though, on just taking action and doing as much as you can, you'll not only burn yourself out, but you'll also find yourself caught up in busy work—doing for the sake of doing.

It's important to balance all of that *doing* with just *being*. Moments where you stop the hustle, breathe, and take time to reconnect with the reasons behind all of that doing.

This can look different from person to person, and even from day to day. For me, "being time" might look like a quick yoga practice before the day starts, catching up on a course I had wanted to take, curling up to read a cheesy romance novel, or even just spending the 30 seconds it takes to walk up the stairs focusing on my breath instead of what I'm going to do at the top of the stairs.

Be Indulgent

Busyness can also lead to an imbalance in how you are spending two of your most precious resources: time and money. The need to rush to get things done means hurried drive-thru meals, throwing on whatever leggings and sweatshirt are closest, quick goodbyes as you drop off one kid and dash to pick up the next…

Focus instead on feeling *indulgent*.

Indulge in a family meal with all the fixings. Indulge in a morning routine to get ready for the day so you walk out of the house feeling confident. Indulge in an extra moment to really feel the hug and appreciate how amazing this person you're raising is.

Granted, things don't always work out that way. It wouldn't be quite fair for me to tell my two-year-old that he has to wait for his breakfast because mama needs to indulge in a morning gua sha routine. But intentionally notice where you can realistically indulge a bit in your day-to-day life.

These indulgences don't have to be big weekend spa getaways, either. Maybe it looks like buying spa-quality towels and spending an extra moment appreciating them when you get out of the shower. Maybe it's setting a timer to take a break every hour to stretch your body and breathe deeply.

These small shifts in your perspective will help break the pattern of continually focusing on *what's next*. Instead, you can spend just a moment appreciating where you are right now and how much you have accomplished already.

The reality is, you are worthy.

What you are doing has a purpose and is impacting the world.

And you don't have to do more, exhaust yourself, or feel overwhelmed in order to prove your value to anyone.

With each inhale you take, you bring in energy and oxygen. Each exhale, though, is neurologically tied to the relaxation response in the brain. You are able to *release*—tension, negative energy, stress—and pause for a single moment before starting the cycle over.

With your next exhale, be intentional about releasing that which is holding you back—anything negative that is keeping you in a cycle of busyness. And then move forward with intention.

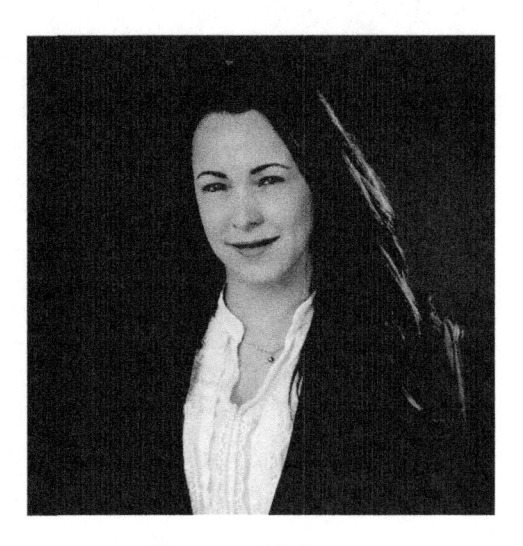

Roxana Valeton

First Person Care Clinic
Chief Executive Officer

https://www.linkedin.com/in/roxana-valeton-01a71456
https://www.facebook.com/Roxy2011leo/about
https://www.instagram.com/rox_valeton/
https://www.tiktok.com/@ladiesturnglobal
https://www.firstpersonclinic.org
https://www.ladiesturn.com

Roxana Valeton is the CEO at First Person Care Clinic, a Federally Qualified Health Center in Nevada providing a variety of services including Primary Care, Dental, Mental Health, Substance Abuse, Pharmacy, and many other services, regardless of the person's ability to pay. Mrs. Valeton serves as a director of the Board of Nevada Primary Care Association, and she is an active member of the National Association of Community Health Centers.

With eight years writing Federal and State grants and 17 years building healthcare businesses, Mrs. Valeton has been able to tap her experience and resources to help vulnerable populations navigate the obstacles of accessible healthcare at a national level. After many years advocating for women's rights and actively creating programs that support mental health awareness she founded LADIES TURN, a secured and professional data driven ecosystem that aims to position ladies in the center of the new global business infrastructure.

TIME TO PULL THE REINS

By Roxana Valeton

We are facing many problems that affect the healthcare arena today in addition to living in uncharted economic territories. I will start by saying that presently, here in the USA, most people have healthcare coverage, but no access. Many hospitals have been forced to close their doors in the last couple of years and counting. There is very limited access to specialty care, and a huge negative gap between the cost of delivering healthcare services and the compensation received by healthcare providers from current covering insurance.

We are living in a new, transformational world, and COVID took it to the next level. For over two years, many people experienced tragedies in their families due to the pandemic, and it is frightening and uncertain what we may discover in the future. We may forget the pandemic, but the way we felt every time we heard about our friends or someone we knew who passed away will stay in our minds forever. Heightened levels of mental health difficulties were commonly reported as well. If you haven't reflected on these experiences, consider doing so. Accept that the change you want to see starts with you.

Some Other Factors Contributing to Today's Healthcare Crisis.

Generally, we don't hear kids or adolescents wanting to become doctors, teachers, or pharmacists anymore. Most of them want to become influencers, social media managers, computer scientists, or get involved in other tech-savvy related jobs. They want to be a part of this new virtual and digital era. I am seeing professionals switching from healthcare related jobs to real estate, IT, AI, and research and development. If you choose your career driven by money, the chances of you changing careers when you are not making the same amount of profit is very likely to happen. This is why I don't believe we have a labor shortage just yet. The healthcare providers are still out there, but they believe nothing is rewarding for them anymore. Health Insurances dictate what medications are covered or not. Even though doctors prescribe the right medication for you, it might not be the one available or covered. Providers are supposed to follow very specific measures that supposedly ensure patients' wellbeing and prevent them from getting ill, even though many are proven not to make any difference in future outcomes. If we analyzed what I just said, the healthcare problems we are facing today are not going anywhere. They will be exacerbated in the future.

How Does the System Work and How Can We Help?

If you understand what supply and demand are, you will realize that if we decide to stop eating fast foods and start eating healthy organic meals, fast food chain companies will have to start changing their menu or they will have to close their businesses. If we stop drinking soda or other soft drinks with excessive sugar added and other unnecessary additives and preservatives, we will have fewer people diagnosed with blood-sugar problems, sleeping disorders, high blood pressure, and allergies, and possibly lower the chances of developing cancer and other chronic diseases—especially if we were not born with them. If we do this, more companies will have to come up with better and healthier products, and as result, hospital visits, doctor's visits, and pharmacy related expenditures will decrease significantly. If our choices change, we will be affecting commodities prices as well, meaning the cost of coffee, meat, grains, and even costs related to energy to name a few.

Since we've been kids, regardless of if you were born into a wealthy family or not, we heard our parents talking about working extra time to save money for a particular situation, and others talking about working far from home because they have to take care of their business or try to expand to a different territory, all for money. Money is the commodity that circulates from person to person to facilitate trade. Lately, I notice more people looking for jobs that allow them to spend more time with their families—jobs with fewer responsibilities, minimal liability, and high reimbursement.

The reality is that we need to allow ourselves to stop thinking about money and stop planning our future for one moment. Our brains will thank us for it. If we take a few minutes daily to meditate and learn about deep breathing techniques, listen, and observe people around us, then we will be more prompt at dealing with overwhelming situations. If you walk daily and engage in your preferred physical activity, your body and mind will get stronger again. If you find the healthy diet of your choice; your skin, your eyes, your liver, your kidneys, and your gut will benefit from it. You will feel energized and happy as a result. By changing our habits we can change our future and the future of our families. We are taking for granted the ability we have to choose what is best for us. We should focus on strengthening our mindset to be able to make worthier decisions.

While interacting with other individuals, nowadays you can sense anger, intolerance, and impatient attitudes. Less personal interactions are making young generations more susceptible to panic attacks, anxiety, and depression because they don't know how to deal with normal life situations they haven't been exposed to before. If you are physically and mentally healthy, you should feel lucky.

Other Recommendations and Resources

- With your healthcare provider's help, write a plan that works for you and try to stick to it.
- Get good-quality sleep on a regular schedule so you feel rested when you wake up.
- Find local farmers in your area that are selling fresh organic foods or a local supermarket that sells certified organic meals.

- Drink plenty of water.
- Learn more about different diet options from professionals. Social media content might not be accurate or updated. I personally listen to Dr. Eric Berg talking about healthy keto and intermittent fasting.
- Read about how smoking can cause frequent urination, and how it is negatively impacting millions of men and women.
- Try to eat foods rich in antioxidants, like: broccoli, cauliflower, carrots, garlic, and onions.
- Ask your healthcare provider how frequently you should empty your bowels. Constipation can lead to several health problems, including cancer.
- Invest in good health insurance coverage that fits your needs. If you can't afford it and you live in the USA, find your local FQHC in your area. They will see you regardless of your ability to pay and will establish a fee for services based on your personal and/or combined household income. You can also try to find free clinics or other resources online.
- Do a wellness exam at least once a year.
- Read about climate change and its impact on your mental and physical health.
- Quit saying "I will die anyways," "I can't stop smoking/or eating dessert," and "exercise isn't for me." I'll tell you a secret: these are all excuses for losers. Take control.

MAKE SURE TO CHECK ALL OF THE ABOVE.

If you want to know more about new healthcare policies and how to get involved, visit: healthcare.gov, SBA.gov, medlineplus.gov, NASHP.gov, or call your local representatives for guidance. If you are a female and want to be actively involved in healthcare initiatives to reduce disparities within communities, or if you want to know about other resources that help accelerate progress toward population health, email: info@ladiesturn.com.

We live unapologetically within a very hypocritical society. Let's take a moment to reflect and act. Tackling difficult health decisions can be the pillar of our preservation. Let's stop feeding the fallacy we live in today. Let's take responsibility for our actions. Let's be the ones who control, not the victims. For a better purpose, let us break this vicious cycle and allow ourselves to change from within. Let's PULL THE REINS.

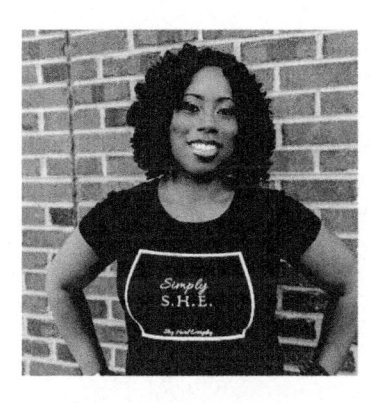

Krystal Vernee'

Simply SHE
Business Coach & Brand Strategist

www.facebook.com/isimplyshe
www.instagram.com/i_simply_she
www.linkedin.com/in/krystalvernee
www.isimplyshe.com
www.slayhardeveryday.co

Krystal Vernee' is a serial womenpreneur, author, speaker, business coach, and brand strategist. She owns Divas & Dolls Fitness, a pole, and sensual dance studio; Cirque Sensual, a sensual aerial dance brand; Simply SHE, a coaching business and podcast and Krystal Vernee' is her personal brand. An engineer by trade, Krystal knew that entrepreneurship was the ultimate goal early in her professional career. She has always been passionate about empowering women, creating a safe space for them to unapologetically be themselves and providing the support they need to transform their passion into profits. Krystal encourages others to tap into her zone of genius through the Simply SHE Podcast and her signature coaching program: The Brand BuildHER BlueprintTM. She teaches coaches and consultants how to build their brand by creating a signature program that attracts their ideal clients.

EXPLORE YOUR INNER DIVA

By Krystal Vernee'

Health and wellness are more than just exercise and healthy eating. When you are healthy holistically, you are healthy mentally, physically, emotionally, and spiritually. As women, we are also at our healthiest when our feminine and masculine energies are balanced. One of the most important lessons I learned a long time ago was that how you feel about yourself as a woman will affect how you move throughout life. It will affect your decision-making, who you choose for friends, what opportunities you pursue, how you let people treat you, literally everything, especially your confidence. After I graduated from college, I reconnected with my now ex-husband and we began dating again. I was admittedly sad and depressed, and our relationship had everything to do with the way that I felt. He knew that I wanted a long-term relationship, and, unfortunately, he manipulated his way back into my heart. He pushed me into a career that I didn't want and constantly made me feel bad about myself. I was stressed, emotionally eating, and I hated the way that I looked because I gained over 60 pounds.

Growing up, I had always struggled with my weight, but I tried to do sports or dance in school to remain active. I tried all my normal methods to lose weight (e.g., going to the gym, dieting, etc.). Something was just different about this time, and I couldn't stay motivated. I couldn't fit in any of my clothes; I would avoid going out with friends that hadn't seen me in a long time, and I just wasn't living life. I had lost touch with my "feminine self" almost completely. Or so I thought. One of my good friends was encouraging me to work out, and she would invite me out all the time to different types of fitness classes. I enjoyed hanging out, but I still hadn't found something that was keeping me working out consistently. One day, she found a deal to try a pole dancing class and the rest is history. I fell in love with the art form and have never looked back. It completely restored my confidence, showed me how my body could move in ways that I never thought possible, and I even started a business teaching other women how to do the same thing. I hope that this chapter will provide insight for women who have and are experiencing the same feelings of not being confident and lost who they are and what they want. I want to shed some light on how getting in touch with my feminine side and *Exploring My Inner Diva* has completely changed my life.

Have you ever felt like you've lost touch with your feminine or sensual side? If we don't nurture this innate part of ourselves as women, we can lose it over time. This is especially true if you're a woman entrepreneur or in a leadership position because it is very easy to slowly gravitate towards more masculine qualities. Leadership is a masculine characteristic, and if you spend most of your time in these spaces, you will naturally start to act more masculine. This doesn't mean that you're turning into a man, but you may find yourself less motivated to dress up, be sexy, walk, or move in a feminine way. You may see femininity as weak, feel more powerful in masculine behavior, neglect self-care, rely on logic rather than intuition, try to control life, etc. Movement awakens your divine feminine or the goddess energy that exists within all of us. Traits of the divine feminine include being intuitive, heart-centered, compassionate, wise, accepting, forgiving, collaborative, etc. It took me years to realize that the reason I was so unhappy and unable to find things that motivated me to be healthier was because I was completely ignoring my need for balance with my feminine side. Sensual dance is movement, and its movement in the most feminine way.

Pole and sensual dance is a fun and creative way to move your body. It increases self-expression and promotes overall well-being. It is a great way to build strength, improve coordination, and boost confidence in an empowering and sexy way. It provides an opportunity to connect with your body and let go of any inhibitions or insecurities. Sensual movement can also serve as a form of release and stress relief. Through this art form, I was able to reconnect with my truest self. It got me through a lot of tough times in my life because I was able to express my emotions through dance and movement. No one around me cared what I looked like or what I had on, how much money I made or didn't make, or what was going on in the world. It was a completely judgement free zone. Once I discovered that it was possible to have this balance for myself, I had to create and hold space for other women to do the same thing. I opened my studio, Divas & Dolls Fitness, so that other women could *Explore Their Inner Diva*, regain their confidence, learn to live a healthier lifestyle, embrace their sensuality and sexuality, and operate in their divine feminine.

I specifically chose "Explore Your Inner Diva" as my company slogan because that is exactly what I did to get to where I am today. I went from being unhealthy, lacking confidence, and being confused about the direction of my life to being CEO of four businesses, living life on my own terms, and being confident in my own skin. When women enter my space, I want them to feel safe, enjoy the community atmosphere, and take what they need to fill their cups. Diva sometimes has a negative connotation, but, in this context, I took the Latin meaning of the word: *goddess*. A diva has self-confidence and self-respect, and carries a certain energy with her that is powerful enough to shift any space she enters. I believe, as women, we explore this part of ourselves our entire lives, as we are always learning, evolving, and transforming.

Exploring your sensual side, especially through movement, is a personal journey and no two are the same. Learning to embrace sensuality in everyday life is important to help you feel confident and empowered as a woman. When you are truly in touch with your sensual side and you embrace *her*, you can then embrace and accept all that you are and becoming. When I was trying to lose weight after college, I was so focused on the weight itself that I didn't pay attention to the rest of me. I didn't check in with myself to see how I was feeling mentally, emotionally, and spiritually. I was concentrating so much on the side effect (e.g., the weight), that I was not addressing the root cause of my issues—not being in touch with myself and who I am. When you just tackle the side effects and don't solve the problem, it reoccurs. This is when I knew I had finally unlocked the mystery behind what I needed to do to live a healthier lifestyle and be the best version of myself. I had to stay in tune with my divine feminine and always be ready and willing to explore my inner diva.

You don't have to take pole and sensual dance classes to *Explore Your Inner Diva* or get in touch with your femininity. These are simple steps that you can take and incorporate into your daily life that will bring you one step closer to embracing your most sensual self:

1. **Set time aside for your self every day that is just for you.** This is not lunch or bathroom breaks, this is time for you to do whatever you want.

2. **Write down what you want to accomplish for the day.** This seems trivial, but when we lack clarity in our minds, even with daily tasks, it can feel more chaotic in our lives.

3. **Incorporate some form of movement into your day.** This can be walking or dancing, but some sort of movement that allows for your feminine qualities to shine (e.g., Yoga, dance fitness, pole dancing, etc.)

4. **Give yourself at least one compliment in the morning.** Negative self-talk tears us down quicker than anyone else ever could. Start to see yourself as the goddess that you are.

5. **Trust your intuition.** "Woman's Intuition" is a real thing! Yes,

logic has a role in life but when something feels off, it typically is. Learn to lean into your intuition when making decisions.

Let the steps above guide you and act as a catalyst for a new journey to tap into the sensual and feminine energies that empower us as women. Whether you choose pole and sensual dance as the means to begin your journey or discover a different way, the key thing is to start, and you will find your way.

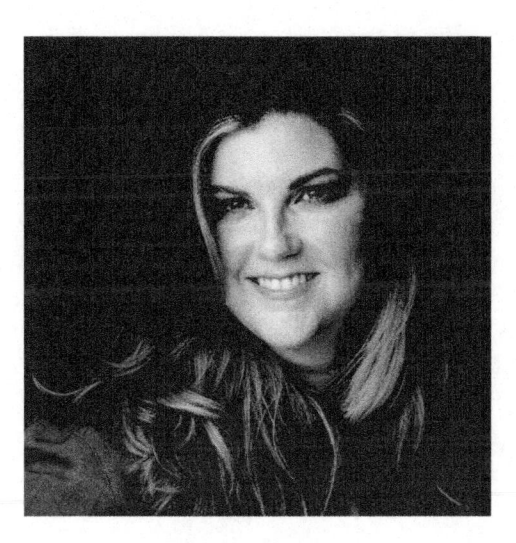

Lauren Weiss

MCHC & MCLC
Female Cycle Advocate

https://www.linkedin.com/in/lauren-e-weiss-female-cycle-advocate-00537a41/
https://www.instagram.com/cyclealign/
https://www.facebook.com/profile.php?id=100046109392085
https://www.cyclealign.com/
http://cyclealignme.com/

Lauren Weiss helps women prosper in life, business, and health by leveraging and understanding the power of their monthly cycle with her exclusive Cycle Align Method™. She has had a lifelong history of hormonal and menstrual cycle mayhem. She went on a quest to understand her body, her cycle, and her innate feminine genius. Along with her deep research and self-awareness, she began to feel energized, creative, and productive again. Her focus shifted to understanding female hormones during the different cycle phases and how women can leverage them to their benefit. Lauren's research and a new understanding of a women's cycle have guided her to be on a mission to debunk the myths, shame, and false understanding of the female body and cycle. She is focused on helping women business leaders lean into their bodies, find harmony and connect with their cycle to enhance their business, life, and relationships.

MIND YOUR FLOW

By Lauren Weiss

Have you ever felt like you are playing Dr. Jekyll and Mr. Hyde? You are one person for one week and then your brain seems to flip a switch and you've transformed into a completely different person the next. I definitely had this issue! I remember my daughter looking up at me one day from her car seat asking me if I was okay. "Yes, sweetie, I'm fine. Why do you ask?" She looks at me with big blue eyes and points at my inside-out shirt. This is where I would insert a face-palm emoji. I promise you are not going insane! There's real science that shows women's brains change throughout the month. I'll explain in this chapter how our brain changes throughout the month as we go through our menstrual cycle and how we can align it with the day-to-day to help our health and wellness.

A study was done in 2018 entitled "Hormonal Influences on Cognitive Function"[1] This study showed through functional Magnetic Resonance Imaging (fMRI) there may be a connection between brain reactivity across the menstrual cycle. This is a lot of scientific jargon, but you may ask: What does this have to do with me? A lot. Certain hormones affect the hippocampus, which helps store memories and social abilities, and the amygdala which dictates emotional regulation. Knowing how certain phases of our cycle and the hormones that are released can affect our brain can help us plan and extend ourselves some grace when we're not at our best.

So let's dive in on what our brain is doing each phase of the month:

1. Menstrual Phase: All hormones are at their lowest point in the body. Serotonin, a brain chemical that is correlated to our

---

[1] Ali, Siti Atiyah, Tahamina Begum, and Faruque Reza. "Hormonal Influences on Cognitive Function." *Malaysian Journal of Medical Sciences* 25, no. 4 (2018): 31–41. https://doi.org/10.21315/mjms2018.25.4.3.

mood, can fluctuate causing us to feel nervous or anxious, irritable, depressed, angry, crying, or become overly sensitive. Knowing that we will be experiencing more unregulated moods or have a harder time with memory we can plan ahead for less strenuous activities and give our brain a break. This is a great time to be gentle with ourselves. Putting extra time and space for pampering experiences will make sure to ease our minds and body allowing us to "fill our cups" so that we can be ready to pour into others for the rest of the month. So go ahead and relax in a luxurious bubble bath or cozy up with a hot cup of your favorite tea and a good book.

2. Follicular Phase: Estrogen is on the rise. Science has shown that estrogen has a therapeutic effect on the nerves and acts as a neuro-protector. It specifically affects the frontal lobe and hippocampus and could be one of the main contributors along with progesterone to aid in neuroplasticity, which essentially is rewiring and changing the brain. This surge of estrogen gives our brains and our bodies energy and revitalization. We might find that we have more desire to be creative and or social. Scheduling time for painting classes, music lessons, or some other creative outlet we desire could take just a pastime into a real skill or craft. Go ahead and grab a friend or loved one and let your inner Picasso or Beethoven out. Doing so feeds your soul and it will feel just as refreshing as rain on a spring day!

3. Ovulation: Estrogen is at its highest point that it will be during this cycle. Estrogen keeps you healthy by encouraging blood flow to the brain, helps decrease inflammation, assists in agility, and memory recall. Estrogen also perks up the amygdala allowing us to sense or better recognize others' feelings or emotions, and the hippocampus gets enlarged which helps us better understand what motivated others. We truly have super

social skills during this time! This extra estrogen also makes you more social and want to be seen! Definitely have those conversations and go to events. Volunteer or reach out and assist those in need.

4. Luteal Phase: Progesterone is at its highest point and hormone levels begin to drop. A 2008 study entitled "Progesterone receptors: form and function in the brain" showed that progesterone has multiple non-reproductive functions specifically with cognition, regulation of mood, mitochondrial functions, myelination (a process forming a protective sheath around nerves to allow information to flow rapidly from one neuron to the next), and could aid in recovery from traumatic brain injuries. It can definitely be defined as a brain neuroprotector! Having this extra progesterone in our brain helps with both verbal processing and visual memory. During this time we may become super aware or have more heightened senses. However, as the progesterone rises we may begin to feel moodier. Why? Progesterone aids the body in producing cortisol. If we are overly stressed and have an excess of cortisol in our bodies (which many do thanks in part to our modern lifestyles) then we will become more irritable and moody. This would be a great time to make sure to grab things that bring us comfort. So snuggle with a loved one or furry friend, watch a favorite show, or sink into a comfy spot to ease our stress.[2]

As you can see with the varying hormonal fluctuations and their effect on the brain, we need to pay attention to our emotions, behavior, and moods, as much as we are to our physical body. By minding our flow

---

[2] Brinton, Roberta Diaz, Richard F. Thompson, Michael R. Foy, Michel Baudry, JunMing Wang, Caleb E. Finch, Todd E. Morgan, et al. "Progesterone Receptors: Form and Function in Brain." *Frontiers in Neuroendocrinology* 29, no. 2 (2008): 313–39. https://doi.org/10.1016/j.yfrne.2008.02.001.

we can increase our mental health and well-being. A person's psychological and emotional well-being should be our top priority! Without our mental health, we can not take care of our basic needs, it can negatively impact our relationships, and it has a direct correlation to our physical health. So often it is hard for humans to know when to make themselves a priority. This problem is an even bigger issue for women, many being caregivers, who are taught through cultural and societal pressures to put themselves last.

So you may be asking at this point "what does my menstrual cycle have to do with my mental health?" It has a great deal of significance! We as women are just incredible and have the gift of morphing and shifting into different versions of ourselves throughout the month. With this gift comes different needs. Knowing our various needs during each phase of our cycle ahead of time allows us to be prepared and cater to our mental health. Do we need to make sure to have more free days during our menstrual week so we can pamper ourselves? Maybe we need to make sure that we are scheduling out dates and fun get-togethers during our ovulation phase so we're not feeling particularly lonely. How about shopping ahead of time so we can make healthier food choices when we are in need of comfort?

Another benefit to being aware of our menstrual cycle and our mental health is that it encourages us to check in daily and listen to our body-mind connection. What does it need today? So often in this modern and busy lifestyle that many of us lead we forget to check in on our needs. Stress is linked to a plethora of health issues, including but not limited to, anxiety, insomnia, gastric issues, and heart disease. An article from The Mayo Clinic[3] encourages setting aside time for

---

[3] Mayo Clinic Staff. "Stress Symptoms: Effects on Your Body and Behavior." Mayo Clinic. *Mayo Foundation for Medical Education and Research*, March 24, 2021. https://www.mayoclinic.org/healthy-lifestyle/stress-management/in-depth/stress-symptoms/art-20050987.

hobbies, practicing relaxation techniques, getting proper physical activity, and of course, spending time with loved ones, all to counteract the effects of stress. How much better would it be to know the optimal time to do each of those activities to maximize the results?

Knowing when to mind our flow so we can get into and stay in the flow of ease in our lives is a great way to become an unstoppable woman in health and wellness! Do you need extra support around knowing your flow or how to mind it? Contact me at bauw@cyclealign.com today! I love supporting women and helping them get in touch with their feminine genius!

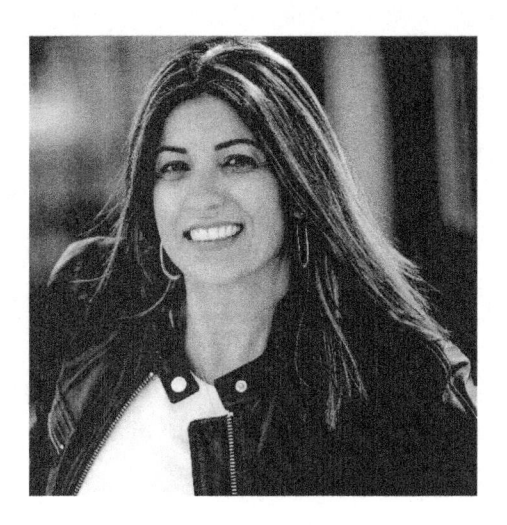

Rita Marrari

Usana Health Sciences Wellness Company
Wellness Coach

http://instagram.com/rmarrari
https://www.facebook.com/rita.marrari.7
https://www.linkedin.com/in/rita-marrari-514b3563
https://ritamarrari.usana.com/

Rita Marrari is a mom of identical twin boys, an entrepreneur, public speaker, dog mom to a feisty golden doodle and a Registered Dental Hygienist based in Toronto, Canada.

Rita has always been passionate about serving others and has always held her health and wellness at the highest of standards.

She always wanted to be a mom, but with a failed marriage at 34, that plan was put on hold. Rita met her true soulmate at 38; having difficulty conceiving she and her new husband embarked on a long and difficult fertility journey.

After five years of unsuccessful IVF treatments she was blessed with her miracle babies at the age of 45!

She had a seamless pregnancy despite being categorized as high risk, the delivery on the other hand was touch and go and traumatic for both momma and babies. Shortly after the babies were born, her health spiralled downwards; postpartum, brain fog, exhaustion, unable to focus; taking care of her precious babies felt impossible!

Rita was able to regain her health and experienced an amazing shift in her energy and overall wellbeing. She felt compelled to share with others the tools that she found and implemented that changed her life! She knew she couldn't possibly be the only mom feeling this way. Rita helps moms make a positive shift in their health, energy, mindset and helps them REIGNITE THE SPARK WITHIN themselves.

REIGNITE THE SPARK WITHIN

By Rita Marrari

The time had come. My emotions were whirling in my head like a tornado, my dream of becoming a momma was about to become a reality. I was scared and excited to finally meet my two miracle babies, the endless injections, years of fertility treatments, dozens of negative pregnancy tests, and the roller coaster of emotions were all spinning in my head.

Okay Rita, you got this, one more push. I gave it all I had, and within a few seconds Baby A slid into the world. The nurses quickly swaddled him and gingerly handed him to my husband to hold. My husband leaned in and whispered "Great job babe, it's 11:48; you have 12 minutes to get baby B out!" What? How? There's no way, I thought to myself! He wanted the babies to have the same birthday, after all, twins have the same birthdays, right? Well, not always.

I was exhausted, there was no way it was going to happen, even if I had the strength and energy at that moment, baby B was not ready. In fact, he was stuck. I could sense things were taking a slight turn for the worst. There was a nervousness and trepidation from the doctors and nursing staff. Baby B was stuck, and I couldn't get him out. After what seemed an eternity, my poor little angel was suctioned out. There was a screeching cry, and the attending nurse snatched him from between my legs and brushed past me briskly. I caught a quick glimpse of his bluish-grey body as my poor little angel whimpered in pain. For months he wore a red disc-shaped bruise on his delicate crown—a reminder of how he was forced into the world.

One last step, push out the placenta and I will finally be able to hold my boys. Well, it wasn't going to be that simple. My placenta did not detach. I could hear whispering amongst the doctors and could see the concern in their faces and their actions. I timidly asked, "What's happening?" and they explained that my placenta did not detach and they needed to remove it. The two interns began ripping at my placenta, buried deep in my abdominal cavity up to their elbows. The organ that provided oxygen and nutrients for my babies had failed me. As they ripped piece after piece, I could hear the ripping of my tissue echo in my ears as each piece plunged into the massive bucket strategically placed under me that was filling up quickly with my blood. They kept ripping so fiercely and violently, that I couldn't bear to see their faces any longer. I turned my head to see my beloved husband, a new dad holding our precious babies in his arms. I faintly whispered, "Please make them stop." The look on his face will forever be etched in my mind. I knew things were not good, and I could feel myself slipping away. From what seemed like another room I heard "I think we got it all." They proceeded to stuff me with meters and meters of gauze to cease the bleeding.

The next afternoon, after refusing a blood transfusion earlier that morning, my obstetrician came to see me with reinforcements. They insisted I have three pints of blood because I had lost so much. I reluctantly gave in and agreed. After being discharged from the hospital, I started experiencing what I thought were normal health issues after having a baby: exhaustion, lack of sleep, brain fog, and anemia. In addition, I had a horrible, persistent cough. One evening while prepping bottles for the boys, I buckled over in a coughing fit which ended in a pile of mushed-up half-digested food. The cough was so violent that I felt a dragging discomfort inside my vagina. It felt like something had dropped. I called my husband into the washroom to have a look. "Ri, it looks like a baby's head. Are you sure there isn't another baby in there!" I had prolapsed, no surprise after having four human arms in my body cavity and carrying two full-term babies weighing in at 6 pounds 7 ounces and 6 pounds 11 ounces. Well, that was not the only reason. After persistent coughs and a second opinion, we were tested for whooping cough. Within 24 hours of the test, I received a call from public health confirming my babies and I had whooping cough and we experienced our first quarantine over the babies' first Christmas and New Year's.

My health was taking a downward spiral fast. The realization that I was a 45-year-old first-time mom came crashing down on me like a ton of bricks. How am I going to take care of my babies? I need to be around for a long time, I want to see them grow up, graduate from university, get married, and I want to see my grandkids. I decided to fight back and regain my health! I started looking for ways to support my health and improve my lifestyle when a friend mentioned cellular nutrition and introduced me to Usana Health Sciences. My cells were starving for essential nutrients, and as I fed my depleted cells I started feeling the benefits. I was still exhausted. I had two babies, how could I not be? But I was feeling the benefits, and my energy levels were increasing. I fell in love with the health shift and the products so much so that I partnered with the company and naturally started sharing with friends and family so I could help make a difference in their lives.

My world revolved, and still revolves, around my babies. As mothers, I think I can safely say our number one priority and focus becomes the health and wellbeing of our children, and I'm sure if asked, every momma would agree wholeheartedly with that statement. I loved my boys more than life itself, but I felt like something was missing. I felt like I lost the Rita I knew before children. My spark had dimmed. I longed for something. I couldn't put my finger on it, but I knew I needed to find my way back to that girl. We all lose our spark at times. I longed for that pulsating, electric feeling in my heart. The guilt for feeling this way weighed heavily on me. How dare I feel this way. I waited so long to have these miracle babies; I endured hardships both physically and emotionally throughout the journey to motherhood.

Being a momma to these beautiful boys should be enough, shouldn't it?

Fast forward to 2020 when I was working as a part-time registered dental hygienist. The office shut down for three months—the entire world shut down! Many faced numerous challenges. The world was shifting, and it was time to adapt to this new world and embrace the change.

I had convinced myself that I couldn't possibly grow my business while having a young family. My husband was very supportive but worked crazy long and unpredictable hours. As training and events shifted to an online platform, I was able to show up and focus on my health and wellness business. I started learning by doing. Was it easy? No, it was definitely a challenge. Technology and I had a turbulent relationship, but I decided to look at this challenge differently, as a way to explore what I was truly capable of. The outcome was incredible, as I discovered strength and power within myself.

As I reflect, I can state benevolently that the only thing that held me back was ME, my belief in myself, and my ability to impact people's lives. My mindset shifted from a fixed mindset to a growth mindset; I was open and ready to take on challenges. I was ready to learn and help others support their health. Now more than ever people were realizing that HEALTH is the true WEALTH! Knowledge became my fuel; the more I learned, the more I presented, and the more events I attended and hosted the more alive I started feeling. I felt a spark ignite inside me and I found my purpose and my passion.

To keep a fire burning, it is necessary to stoke the fire by adding fuel and oxygen. I had ignited the spark within, but what could I do to keep the fire burning bright and keep it from dying out? You need to set time aside for personal development. Personal development is a vital part of an individual's growth and progression. Personal development allows you to explore areas of self-improvement, master skills, and feel self-fulfilled. The more I learned and grew the more I wanted to learn and grow. I was hungry like a newborn hungering for milk.

My community was a huge motivation and factor. I was surrounded by positive, like-minded individuals who supported me, inspired me, and cheered me on. The way I started feeling empowered and confident was like adding lighter fuel to my spark. It began to roar with hot, fierce flames. The more I surrounded myself with positivity, the more my tolerance for negativity became negligible, and I noticed more positivity, goodness, and opportunities presenting themselves.

Don't be afraid to step out of your comfort zone, for on the other side of that fear and trepidation is the greatest growth.

Never say no to an opportunity because risk is better than regret!

Have faith that God and the Universe are leading you in the right direction.

Take small steps. Small steps lead to big changes.

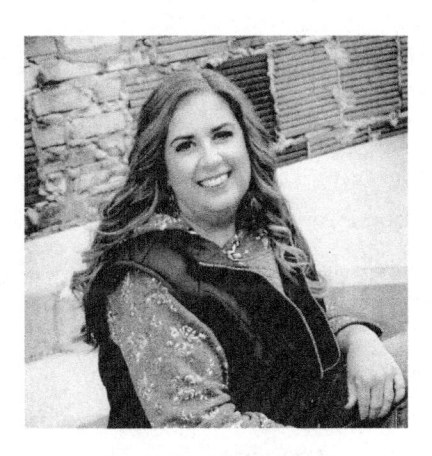

Kim Rendon

Live&Thrive Wellness, LLC
Registered Dietitian / Certified Health Coach

https://www.linkedin.com/in/kim-rendon-824073218/
https://www.facebook.com/kimcoaches2020
https://www.instagram.com/livethrive_wellness
https://www.livethrivewellness.com

Kim Rendon is a registered dietitian and certified lactation specialist. She has been an RD for 30 years, working with pregnant and breastfeeding women and their children. In addition to working as an RD, she started her own integrative health coaching business.

She is on a mission to educate the world about perimenopause and menopause. She wants it to become the norm to talk about it and that women don't have to hide and feel like they are going crazy or broken. Kim has an advanced certification in hormone health and gut health. She is a self-declared science geek who loves talking about gut bugs and how they affect hormones.

She is a boy mom who dealt with puberty during perimenopause, and everyone has lived to talk about it. Now that her boys are grown, Kim likes to spend her spare time traveling and sitting on a beach somewhere warm.

BECOME AN AGELESS GODDESS

By Kim Rendon

Close your eyes and take a few deep breaths. I want you to look into the future to the 90-year-old version of yourself. How does that 90-year-old you feel about the life you have lived? Is it the life you want to have lived?

I had my boys in my mid-30s, which meant I was going through perimenopause at the same time as they were going through puberty. Perimenopause is just puberty in reverse. You can only imagine the raging hormones and moodiness that was in that household.

Both boys were active and three-sport athletes. During this time, I worked full-time, ran them to practices and games, was on the Christian education board at church, was vice president of the athletic boosters, and ran concession stands. I was tired and overwhelmed. Some days, I didn't know what direction I was going. There were times that meals were thrown together for a quick meal or eaten on the run. Think hot dogs, popcorn, and Mountain Dew in the bleachers of whatever sporting event we were at.

Along with the overwhelm and the exhaustion, depression began to happen. Some days felt like I couldn't keep it together and couldn't think straight. I experienced brain fog or forgot what I was saying in the middle of it all. I figured this was just life.

Then my oldest left for the Marine Corps, and my husband and I separated. The depression worsened, and I began to self-medicate with cookies and junk food. I gained a lot of weight and began to hate myself for it.

Add to that the hot flashes and waking in the night so hot I couldn't get back to sleep, and I was a hot mess. I didn't associate what was happening with the hormonal fluctuations that they were.

As I started researching more about menopause, I realized what was happening was normal, and I was ok.

Menopause is not talked about much. We may joke about "the change" and giggle at the woman having a hot flash, but we suffer in silence. Now, I've made it my mission to educate the world about menopause and to make it ok to talk about it. For goodness' sake, do you see menopause being talked about on TV like erectile dysfunction is? **NO**

So, let's talk about perimenopause and menopause.

What is perimenopause? It wasn't a word that I had heard until I started researching menopause. Perimenopause is the time leading up to menopause, the transition. Menopause is technically one day. The day you have gone 12 months without menstruating. After that, it becomes post-menopause.

Perimenopause typically starts in the mid-40s but can be as early as the mid-30s and lasts, on average, eight to 10 years. Diet and lifestyle can contribute to the age at which perimenopause starts. So, if you are reading this and thinking, "I'm not there yet," it will happen, and the sooner you start taking care of yourself, the easier the process can be. The average age of menopause is between the ages of 49 and 51.

Induced menopause is an early or sudden onset due to surgical removal of the ovaries, chemotherapy or radiation, and premature ovarian failure.

How do you know perimenopause has begun? We all know the typical hot flashes and night sweats, irregular periods, low libido, mood swings, and vaginal dryness or painful intercourse, but did you know there are around 40 symptoms of menopause?

Just a few of them are...

- Heart palpitations
- Joint and muscle pain

- Flare-ups of arthritis
- Worsening of chronic illnesses
- Digestive issues: gas, bloating, indigestion, constipation, or diarrhea
- Hypoglycemia
- Headaches or migraines
- Incontinence
- Loss of muscle tone
- Memory challenges and brain fog
- Anxiety, depression, and panic attacks

If you are experiencing any of these, don't just assume it is from perimenopause. Always follow up with your healthcare provider.

Those tiny little messengers we call hormones are what cause this train wreck, and when I say hormones, I'm talking about more than just estrogen and progesterone. There is testosterone, thyroid, cortisol, and glucose involved. There is a fine balancing act between them. One little change throws off at least one other hormone.

Perimenopause begins when progesterone begins to decrease, leaving us in a state of estrogen dominance. Progesterone is our feel-good, chill-out hormone. Estrogen dominance is where many of the symptoms begin.

Women all experience it differently. Why are you having terrible hot flashes when your best friend hasn't had any issues? Many times, it comes down to diet and lifestyle, but did you know that the health of your gut matters, too? Your gut health affects hormonal balance.

So, what's a girl to do?

Diet:

1. Eat enough calories - When you deprive your body of calories, it puts you in a state of stress. Eat the right balance of

macrobiotics: fat, protein, and carbohydrates.

2. Eat healthy fats - Yes, I said eat fat. We need fat for hormone production, brain function, energy, and the protection of vital organs. Omega 3 fatty acids are essential for us, but our bodies are unable to produce them. The Omega 3 fats lower the risk of getting chronic diseases such as heart disease, arthritis, and cognitive conditions. They can also reduce inflammation which can lead to autoimmune diseases and even depression. You can find them in fatty fish like salmon and mackerel, walnuts, coconut oil, and avocados.

3. Eliminate processed foods and sugar – In a world of highly processed, nutrient-deficient, sugar-ladened foods, we are slowly killing ourselves. Inflammation is one of the side effects of a processed food lifestyle. Inflammation damages your heart, brain, and your gut.

4. Choose an anti-inflammatory diet lifestyle - The top pro-inflammatory foods are gluten, corn, soy, dairy, sugar, and processed food. When you begin to eliminate these foods, your body can begin to heal itself. All bodies are unique, so you may be able to tolerate some of these foods or eat them occasionally.

5. Gut health - Eat or drink fermented foods, which are good sources of probiotics, or take a probiotic supplement. Probiotics are good gut bugs. Our poor diet, the use of antibiotics and other medications, alcohol, stress, and inadequate sleep allow the bad gut bugs to take over the good.

6. Decrease your toxin load - There are toxins everywhere, in our foods, water, plastic, cookware, and your body care items. Many of them can act like a hormone or block your body from using or producing them.

Lifestyle:

1. Decrease stress – Your body perceives being chased by the tiger, running late for work, or not eating the right diet as stress, and responds the same way to them all. It shuts down many of the body's functions to protect itself for survival. Stress produces the hormone cortisol. When we are in a continual state of stress, it causes inflammation in the body and the gut and limits the production of progesterone and testosterone.

2. Meditate – Meditation bridges the connection between mind and body. Some of the benefits of meditation include decreasing stress, decreasing depression, decreasing inflammation, increasing immunity, reducing blood pressure, and improving sleep, to name a few.

3. Journal - There are many reasons to journal. It can help you get clarity. It helps to get the mental shit, as I call it, out. It helps you to learn to listen to yourself, it can help alleviate stress, and manage depression and anxiety. Make it a gratitude journal. It's hard to be negative when you are busy being grateful.

4. Sleep - Getting seven to nine hours of good quality sleep is so important. This is where your body can heal itself. Set up a bedtime routine to help prepare your body for sleep and turn off electronics at least an hour before bed.

5. Deal with past traumas – There is a mind, body, and soul connection. We hold unresolved trauma in our bodies that can manifest not only emotionally but physically.

6. Exercise – Move your body, getting some sort of physical activity most days of the week. Do what makes you feel good. If that means turning up the music and dancing, taking a walk

through the park, or doing Yoga, do it. Do low-intensity workouts along with strength training.

Tired of being tired, tired of the depression, and tired of the weight, I started my own health journey. It has been a slow process, making small changes because our "critter" brains don't like change and try to hold us back even though we know that making these changes is the best for us.

When I look at the energy I have, how much clearer my brain is, and the weight loss without even trying, I'm grateful for the changes that I made even if they did feel like a sacrifice at the time. Do I still have a ways to go? Yes, but that 90-year-old me is living her best life.

Don't look at this stage in life as the beginning of the end, but as the beginning of a new stage in life. Become the ageless goddess you are born to be.

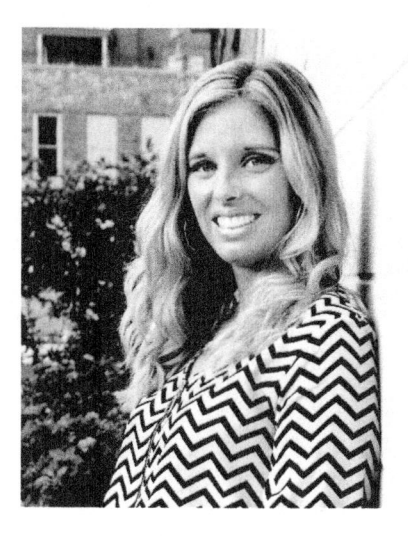

Nicole Curtis

Executive Assistant to the CEO of She Rises Studios

https://www.facebook.com/nicolecurtissherisesstudios
https://www.instagram.com/nicolecurtis_sherisesstudios/
https://www.facebook.com/groups/sherisesstudioscommunity
https://www.sherisesstudios.com/

Speaker, Author, and Mentor. Nicole is a tenacious woman geared to serving and helping women grow, elevate and succeed in life and in business. Nicole's mission is to not only educate and empower women, she specializes in building true authentic professional relationships with women all over the world. Nicole loves to support and guide women in business to become more visible worldwide and she is a mental health advocate for moms with struggling children.

A MENTAL HEALTH "CHECK IN" LIST FOR MOMS WITH STRUGGLING TEENS

By Nicole Curtis

I am the mother of a teen girl who has suffered from major depression and anxiety over the last five years. As a family, we have dealt with two partial hospitalizations and one hospitalization admission, numerous suicide attempts, cutting incidents, and run aways. We've attended years of counseling and tried many different medication regimens to try to help. I've been screamed at, lied to, and have had countless sleepless nights.

I know that for some of you mamas your situation and circumstances are different from mine, and that is okay, but the one thing we have in common is the heartache we feel for our babies. It is painful watching our teens suffer when all we want to do is "fix" it for them. We find ourselves wishing they could be "normal" teens. We so desperately want them to feel happy. We encourage them to socialize and find friends. We want them to know that they are loved and that they matter—that their life matters!

Being a supportive mom to a teen who struggles with her mental health, I have learned just how important it is that you protect your own mental health. I know that when you're trying to help, support, encourage and assist in all the things it is easy to put yourself and your own needs on the back burner. I get it!! I did this for years and it wasn't pretty. I want to provide you with a mini guide that offers you a mental check-in list which you can use every day to help you protect your mental health. I wish someone would have said or given me this guide early on.

There is an extreme lack of information available outside of the common mental health brochures that are specifically centered around providing mental and emotional support to moms (parents or caregivers) that have teens (or children) that struggle with mental health, and I want to be that source of information for you. I want you to not only be the best you you can be, but I want to help you show up in the best state of mind you can for them. In sharing my mental health "Check-In" list for Moms, my hope is that you use it and that it becomes just as useful to you as it has for me.

Mental Health "Check In" List for Moms With Struggling Teens:

It Is Okay Not To Be Okay:

I want you to permit yourself to feel! No matter how hard it hurts or how sad it feels. Helping your child through unimaginable things is scary and downright terrifying. I know that in the moment it is easy for us moms to put our "game face" on, and sometimes we have to just get through the circumstances or episode that is occurring and that is okay. Sometimes, having our teen see us be strong offers them a sense of safety and security. I get that, but when things settle down or you find yourself consumed by so many emotions you got to let that out, mama! You can't keep it buried inside of you, otherwise, it is going to eat away at you. You need to process what has happened, or what is happening to be your best self and continue supporting your teen.

This mental health journey your child is on is hard, terrifying, and is downright ugly. What has helped me process my emotions during our journey is writing down all that I am feeling! For me, being able to see it on paper and read it helps me be consciously aware of what is happening internally. Oftentimes when I am doing this, I find myself either ugly crying or feeling a sense of anger, and that is okay. It is okay to feel sad, angry, fearful, tired, and hurt! Heck, it is okay if you need to take a step back at times and give yourself space to regroup and process. Go for a drive, take a walk, or go visit a trusted friend. This doesn't make you a bad mom, it makes you a courageous mom. Take time for yourself to breathe!

The point is: yes, there are times when we need to be strong, but don't let that strength begin to lie to you. Don't let it consume you so much that you begin to believe you can't ask for help or support yourself. You are not in this alone!! I have joined many support groups and reached out to other moms who are going through the same thing.

You Can't "Fix" It:

I can't tell you how many times I have gotten angry at the fact that sometimes, no matter how much I offered my help, it has gotten thrown back in my face. How many nights—and days, let's be honest—that I have cried because I wished I could fix the situation my teen is battling, but the reality is I can't. The "fixing" has to come from them.

There have been countless times when I found myself spinning my wheels trying to help and support them only to find us right back to the same place, or worse three steps back. I started to internalize this, and I began blaming myself. I blamed myself for what was happening to my daughter. I thought that I must be a bad mom, or that I messed up in raising her. I had to realize that I can offer as much help and support as I can to her, and if it isn't reciprocated that isn't something I can fix. I know we moms always want the best for our children and that isn't a bad thing, but when they start to reject you or the help you offer please don't let it make you believe that you are a failure. They are hurting and suffering and sometimes when they lash out or decide they don't want to continue taking meds, go to counseling, or are done with any sort of help no matter how hard you "beg" them to continue, you are not to blame.

Where Do I Go From Here:

I have often found myself wondering: What do I do now? Where do I go from here? These questions come up whenever my advice or assistance is no longer receptive to my daughter. At first, I would freak out because this "rebellion" scared the crap out of me. I was paranoid that if I didn't help or provide something, then it was going to have negative effects, or that if she no longer wanted my help then everything was for sure going to come crashing down. It took a while to conclude that the "rebellion" of these things was on me. Sometimes, she actually needs to have a break. And trust me, there were times I over-stressed so many programs, information, activities, etc because I wanted to help, but it actually stressed her out more in the end. I learned that it is okay to take a step back, and that if she didn't want my advice or assistance I shouldn't overreact and think the worst. Instead, when these times happened it allowed time for us to pause and adjust. It created an opportunity for us to communicate with one another. It opened the door for her to tell me how she is feeling so I could come alongside her differently, instead of how she often put it: "pushy" or "naggy."

Stop walking on Eggshells:

Boy oh boy is this a biggie! I don't know about you, but this one has been the hardest one for me not to do! With all of the hard, scary, and heavy stuff we have gone through as a family and all of the things I have personally witnessed, separating my feelings and thoughts has been a challenge. I find myself oftentimes stressing about how the day is going to go and how to approach or hold a conversation with her so I don't "set her off." How do I go about disciplining her? I've even been scared to say NO to her! I was afraid of what I might get back in return. When I am walking on eggshells with her, I notice I treat my other teen differently. I am a lot stricter and sometimes put a higher expectation on him than his sister, which then causes tension between our relationship as well as a family unit. I share this vulnerability to show you I am a real mom who is trying her best to navigate motherhood. If you, too, find yourself doing these same things, then this is when it is so important for us parents to parent our children versus trying to be their friends. There needs to be a certain level of respect, trust, and authority. I can't let the manipulation of my daughter control my every move, especially with how I am to parent. I had to learn to stand my ground and stand up for myself. I can't control her reactions, but I can control mine. I can't control what she does or says,

but I can control what I do and say! I can't live in fear of the what ifs and the unknowns. I have to show up as my best self every day and doing daily mental check-ins on my thoughts and pausing to take three deep breaths before any words come out of my mouth has been a huge help! :)

I dedicate this chapter and send my love to all the mamas who are doing their best to help and support their struggling teens, and to my beautiful baby girl, I love you so very much!

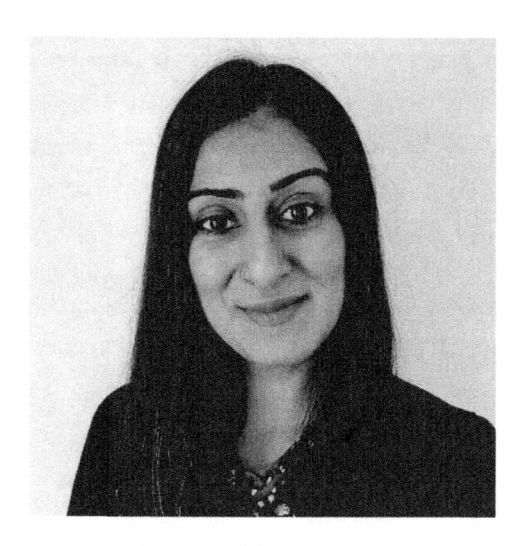

Divya Chandegra

Chit Ltd
Life & Wellness Soul Guide

https://www.instagram.com/divya.chandegra/
https://www.facebook.com/Life-and-Wellness-with-Divya-115873590689176
https://www.divya-chandegra.com
https://www.divya-chandegra.com/subscribe

Divya Chandegra is a life and wellness soul guide. Her mission in life is to empower parents and professionals to heal their limiting childhood beliefs and subconscious blocks. She guides them to focus on their inner child, generational patterns, mindset reprogramming, self-love, and unconditional love.

Divya is passionate about seeing her clients transform by releasing repeated behavior patterns through conscious decision-making to avoid passing trauma on to future generations!

She truly believes through personal experience of healing complex trauma that the key is in improving the connection with Self first. In turn, saving children from 20-30 years of exposure to generational wounds and societal programs that impact their connections, careers and self-belief systems that resurface for healing later in life.

Subscribe for free access to her Understanding Your Inner Child mini-course and Unblock Your Self masterclass to begin your transformation journey today!

ATTRACT FULFILLMENT AND SUCCESS THROUGH BALANCE AND SELF-LOVE

By Divya Chandegra

The Seasoned Over-Giver

I was raised in a very giving family. After spending over 30 years giving my time, attention, and energy to the needs of others, I realised that I was becoming frustrated and resentful. My 'giving' was no longer authentic and pure the way my parents intended to raise us. This was not who I wanted to be.

I watched my parents give freely to others at the expense of their wellbeing. I was raised with the same programming, and I no longer wanted to play the game that I'd been playing for decades—putting the needs of others before my own.

Boundaries and Balance

I lived with the inability to and a fear of saying 'no' to others, because of what they would think of me. So, I'd take on way too much in every aspect of my life, overcommitting to things and never quite finding balance. Giving, doing, and ensuring I didn't let people down was causing an imbalance in my mental, physical, emotional, and spiritual wellbeing. I didn't know about healthy boundaries, because I didn't know *my Self* and because I believed that if I couldn't give to others, then I wasn't worthy in my own right.

Not being able to express my Self, not being able to say 'no,' and not being able to identify my needs and communicate them in my personal and professional (male-dominated) environment was debilitating. I had to exercise control in every aspect of my life to keep my anxiety at bay. I was holding on to all of the emotional tension in my energetic and physical body. And it didn't feel good. I was unhappy, even if it appeared like I had everything under control. Something had to change.

Wellness and Self-Care

> *"It's all about falling in love with yourself...rather than looking for love to compensate for a self-love deficit."*
> —Eartha Kitt

My breakthrough moment arrived when I realised that I was looking for others to love me unconditionally, and yet I wasn't loving my Self in that way. I grew up in an environment of conditional love, modelled not only by my family but in our culture by society, the fairy tales, movies, books, and the expectations we place on ourselves and others.

If I spoke and behaved in a particularly idealised way, especially as a British Indian woman—only then would I be loved and accepted by the world around me. The impact this had on my personal and professional connections meant that I was constantly seeking validation from outside sources. The belief I was reinforcing was that if I met *their* expectations, if I was 'perfect,' then I would be good enough, valued and worthy.

The Impact of Our Childhood

The issue I had with this ingrained belief about my Self is that it didn't feel true to my Soul. How could I truly love, care, be understanding and accepting of others, if I couldn't be that for my Self? I grew up in an environment where I struggled to express my Self, and I didn't know how to identify my own needs.

I never learned how to process my emotions, let alone actually allow myself to experience them. If something 'good' happened, it was about being better instead of appreciating and celebrating the success or experiencing joy in the present. I compartmentalised any anger, frustration, sadness, and fears by putting on a mask, and I became really good at it over the years.

The Imbalances

In childhood, I was taught to be there for others, to be of service, and to do what others (elders, our customs, culture, our gender roles, and tradition) expect. With that, the pain, deep dissatisfaction, and resentment built up and started impacting my mental, emotional, spiritual, and physical Self. I had to find a way to reduce the noise and to hear the call of my Soul. I needed to identify my needs and learn to give to my Self with love, compassion, acceptance, and understanding.

At 17 years, I had chronic back pain that the doctors couldn't diagnose. I couldn't sit, lay down or stand, I hardly ate and was in excruciating pain 24/7. I now know that it was an imbalance in my chakras from storing emotional trauma that caused the energetic blocks in my physical body.

Throughout childhood, I was taught to focus on my career and finding a partner. I was in my final year at university and my parents were already talking to me about getting married. How could I prioritise these two key aspects of my life, when I didn't know how to bring my Self to balance?

I needed to learn how to give to my Self in a healthy way. How could I possibly have honest, balanced, and loving connections with others when I was unable to show up for my Self and understand my needs with honesty, non-judgement, and self-love?

Connection With Others

> *"If you don't love yourself, nobody will. Not only that, you won't be good at loving anyone else. Loving starts with the self."*
> —Wayne Dyer

Sometimes, we're so busy in our own minds that we forget to be present and create a safe space for others, so that they can communicate openly and without fear of judgement. The more we practise this, the more we can build a realness in our connections that exceed the limits of societal expectations, our fears, generational, and gender stereotypes.

I lived most of my life like this—in fear of being judged. I then inflicted these programs onto others. I judged others based on *my* perceived conditional values even though they didn't feel true to me. I expected more and better from them, because I never felt good enough as I was. As an adult, I explored and studied my unmet childhood needs, and I *practised* and reprogrammed my Self to believe and know that I am good enough, irrespective of the things that I do or don't do for others. My validation of Self no longer relies upon seeking approval from others, and I'm freeing my Self, so that I can guide my loved ones to do the same!

Our Impact on Others

We have to decide the role we want to play in the lives of our families, friends, and future generations. Do we want them to be raised thinking that connections with others are conditional? Or do we want to nurture them to practise giving to themselves, so they're not dependent on others to fulfill their unmet needs?

Our ability to truly and authentically connect with others rests on our ability to learn who we are—to learn our needs as adults and to give to ourselves first. When we're able to do this, we can come to our connection with others with pure intentions, a deep understanding, vulnerability, and courage to defend *our* real values and principles, instead of those we've been led to believe since childhood.

Success and Self-Growth

> *"Your work is to discover your world and then with all your heart give yourself to it."*
> —Buddha

Learning your Self and what you stand for as an adult allows you to identify what success means to *you*. My programming led me to believe that success is financial wealth or being married with children because of the scarcity mindset and traditional expectations placed on me from childhood. I had to teach my Self that success is in other things... it's in celebrating when I've been able to bring my Self to balance after a long week. It's in the ability to identify my needs when my energy is in flux. It's in being able to set healthy boundaries for my best and highest good, instead of feeling guilty for saying 'no.' It's in unlearning my limiting subconscious childhood beliefs and learning who I truly am. It's in living in my truth and serving my purpose, now that I know who *I* am.

Creating the Life You Desire

You have a gift in life to create the reality you want and choose to live. You have to choose what you want in this life, make a plan, and take action to get what you want. Most of it will reveal itself to you when you learn to build a connection with your Self and reprogram your limiting childhood beliefs. You'll realise that you can achieve anything when you learn to bring your Self to balance.

When you're living in your truth and continue to work through your layers of programming, you'll see that the only consistent thing in life is that you're *always* growing.

Choosing to Love Your Self First

If you desire fulfilment and success in life, focus on learning your Self to avoid placing expectations on others to fulfill your unmet needs and unhealed wounds. This enables you to connect through acceptance, understanding, and unconditional love for Self and others, in a balanced way.

My mission is to be of service to our community, future generations, and our environment through conscious living.

My eBook, *Success Starts with Self: 35 Must-Read Articles to Set You Up for Long-Term Success* focuses on Wellness & Self-Care, Connection & Relationships, Success & Growth, and is available for purchase for a nominal fee through my website www.divya-chandegra.com/books

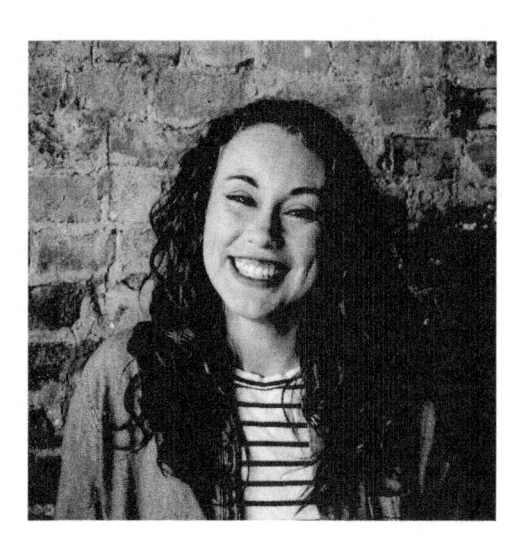

Brandi Kepley

Founder of the Unfinished Grace Community
Podcaster | Blogger | Arbonne Consultant

www.Instagram.com/unfinishedgrace
https://www.linkedin.com/in/brandi-kepley-762b09215/
https://www.facebook.com/groups/883784352340904/?ref=share_group_link&exp=93fa
www.unfinishedgrace.com
www.brandikepley.Arbonne.com

Brandi is a wife, dog mom, Arbonne consultant, blogger, and podcaster. When she isn't working, you can find her reading at a local coffee shop or hiking with her husband and dogs.

Her ministry, the Unfinished Grace community, exists to identify with and encourage those struggling with mental health issues and stigmas. She is passionate about stigmas within family units and within the church, ending the cycle of burnout, and promoting a healthy lifestyle with natural products.

Brandi has struggled with anxiety and depression for many years, but encountered a serious mental health crisis in the spring of 2021. She and her husband decided the best course of action was for her to immediately quit her job and find part-time work from home. God then laid it on her heart to share her story with others, and in a few short months, the Unfinished Grace ministry was born.

UNFINISHED HEALING

By Brandi Kepley

I thought that was it. I thought I was finished. I didn't think I could take one more breath, let alone one more day.

I felt so trapped inside my mind. The uncontrollable panic just wouldn't stop. The weight was too heavy. I couldn't breathe, couldn't move, couldn't keep going—and I didn't want to.

You know, it's true what they say—sometimes you have to hit rock bottom to realize that God is the rock at the bottom.

That's where I was: rock bottom.

I've struggled with anxiety and depression for as long as I can remember, even though I didn't fully realize what it was early on. But this was it, this was the end. Or so I thought.

I was 22 years old and working my butt off in a retail leadership position that I should have been making much more for. This was the third job in a row that I had held where I was overworked, underpaid, and underappreciated. I had felt the looming dread start to creep in before and tried to fix the issue by changing the scenery, but it was the same everywhere I went. The external factors were increasingly worsening, but the real root of the problem was internal; I couldn't escape it.

I should have been over the moon. I had graduated with my bachelor's degree, gotten married to my high school sweetheart, bought a home, and had amazing friends and two loveable pups that I adored. But there was still an empty, black hole in my chest.

My husband knew things weren't all rosy, but I was trying to hide the scary from him. I knew he would worry. He had a health condition that was affected by extreme stress. Sleep deprivation, exhaustion, and intense stress can cause those with epilepsy to go into seizures, and those grand mal seizures are unbearable. There's nothing like holding your spouse's head while he violently convulses, foaming at the mouth, face and lips turning blue, unable to breathe, and then calling an ambulance and sitting in the emergency room with him all day because he won't stop vomiting. I developed PTSD from these multiple instances. Our individual medical conditions only add to the stress of the other. His epilepsy increasing my anxiety, my anxiety triggering his epilepsy- it's a chaotic cycle.

But at some point, I had to tell him how bad it was. I vowed on our wedding day not to hide even the ugliest parts of me, so this was it. I told him how bad it was with tears rolling down my face. "I need you to take me to the doctor," I sobbed. "I can't do this anymore. I don't want to live anymore."

After an extremely long day of doctors and counseling appointments, after prayer and consideration, we decided together that it was best that I immediately resign from my corporate position. My number one priority was now staying alive. We didn't know how, but God would take care of the rest.

It's A Journey

My perfectionist, fast-tracked brain had a hard time stopping. I had to contribute somehow. I had to have something to do, but my personality has always been to overfill my plate. I had never felt "enough," and that was a big roadblock.

The worst part, though, was telling others. I've always worried too much about what others think—don't we all? One of my biggest fears was being seen as less than, weak, or lazy. The expectation was to get a degree, go to work, and fake it until you make it. Even if you weren't really happy, well, that was just life. No one really likes their job.

But you should at least want to live, right? Things shouldn't be this bad.

I had no idea what I wanted to do with my life. I knew I wanted to be happy, have a family, and serve Jesus. That was all I knew. I never imagined I would do full-time ministry.

I always felt that I had something to say, something to teach. I often imagined myself being a speaker. Why, though, I'm not sure, because I hated speaking in front of others. And yet, this little part of me still craved that someone would see me and listen to what I had to say because it was important.

I was anxious and introverted and thought no one could ever actually learn anything from me. I thought about adding a comment or asking a question in school or Bible studies, but people would probably just laugh at me and think I was stupid. What made perfect sense in my mind would be a wreck in theirs.

For as long as I can remember I had a little voice in my head telling me to keep quiet, but maybe now, I thought, I should give it a chance. I mean at this point, what did I have to lose? I was already at the end of the road—or what feels like it at least.

But God's Grace

I decided it was time to say "yes" to that not-so-little inkling I had been feeling for some time. It was time to stop saying "that's definitely not for me," stop giving God borders, and just see what God would do. Sometimes the truth hurt, but that same truth could also save someone else's life. That made it worth it.

While I felt unworthy and incapable of writing and producing content that would encourage others, I remembered that God doesn't call the equipped but equips the called. "Okay, God. Here I am. Use me."

I started writing, and it all just flowed out. It can be painful to relive trauma and emotions, but it can also be so restorative at the same time. After many hours of writing, creating a website, researching marketing, networking, and praying for guidance and clarity, I launched my blog sharing my journey and growth with mental health: Unfinished Grace.

God laid that title on my heart because He was constantly showing me that He wasn't finished with me yet. He was also teaching me what grace really looked like on a daily basis.

I felt some dark and scary things. BUT GOD'S GRACE.

I thought depression and anxiety were all there were. BUT GOD'S GRACE.

I cut my arm with a knife just to feel something. BUT GOD'S GRACE.

I didn't want to keep going. BUT GOD'S GRACE.

I thought I was done. BUT GOD'S GRACE.

His grace was always enough, but I had to let it be enough.

Keep Going

After a few months of blogging and networking, I felt God calling me to start a podcast. I had thought that a podcast would be a great addition to the ministry someday, but I thought I had to be much further down the road. Then a friend told me about her podcast and how easy it was to set up. I decided that it was time. We aren't ever really "prepared," so we might as well just jump in!

I have been blown away by how God has used the Unfinished Grace podcast! I didn't think anyone would want to be interviewed for the show and share their own story, but they have! I didn't think anyone would listen and share the episodes with their community, but they have!

On my journey, I discovered Arbonne, a wellness company that transformed my health from the inside out. I have learned how important every aspect of wellness is and how every system in the body works together. I am constantly in awe of God's handiwork and the tools He has given us to live our best life.

This is just the tip of the iceberg. My story is also woven with emotional abuse, trauma, and so much more. One chapter could never hold someone's entire story, so if this resonated with you I would love to connect. But, since I have to wrap it up, I want to leave you with a few encouraging thoughts.

Final Thoughts

Remember that you are not defined by your thoughts and feelings.

A lot goes into mental illness: chemical imbalances, spiritual warfare, mindset, lack of vital nutrients, lack of self-care, external stresses, physical trauma- the list goes on and on. Be patient with yourself during this process. Every day is a new day with new opportunities.

You have options when it comes to what you allow in your body. Choose wisely. The chemicals in your products will affect every ounce of your health so educate yourself.

I am a firm believer that God can miraculously heal through prayer. But I also believe that He has given us tools, such as medication and therapy, that can be monumental in our journeys.

Community is a necessity. We were created for relationships. Don't do life alone.

Nothing changes the way Jesus sees you. His greatest works are revealed in our weaknesses (2 Corinthians 12:9).

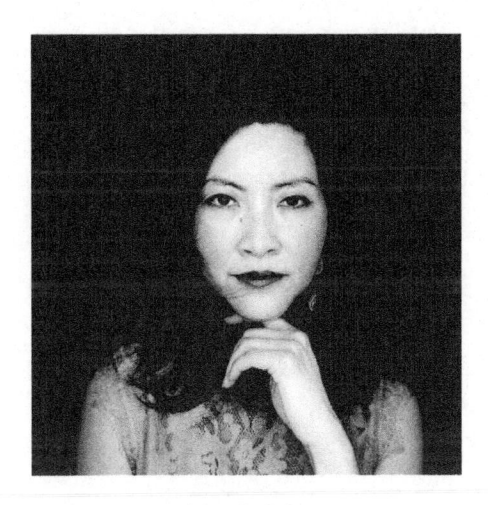

Minh Vu

Endotransformation
Holistic Endometriosis and/or Infertility Coach

https://www.instagram.com/endotransformation/
https://www.linkedin.com/in/endotransformation/
https://www.facebook.com/groups/endotransformation
https://endotransformation.com/

Minh Vu, authority in firsthand experience with holistic health in endometriosis and infertility. CEO and founder of Endotransformation, she empowers women diagnosed with endometriosis and/or infertility to advocate for their own health.

Personally diagnosed with Stage 4 endometriosis and infertility, Minh advocated for her own health by implementing a holistic path that liberated her from endometriosis pain and symptoms. Miraculously, despite all odds, she naturally conceived twin boys!

As a Holistic Endometriosis and Infertility Coach, she curates journeys that transform women's lives. The 'MODERN DAY LIBERATED WOMAN,' she empowers you to liberate feminine power from endometriosis and infertility trauma to awaken your divine true self.

When not immersed in her mission, Minh enjoys her loved ones and savors sacred moments in nature! Since becoming a mother, the only resolutions Minh has stuck to is swapping skinny jeans for mom jeans and relishing in her liberation. She's never been happier!

LIGHT AND THE PROTECTIVE WARRIOR

By Minh Vu

Lesson #1: Be Your Own Health Advocate (Narrator: Minh Vu)

At 33 years old, Tom and I seriously tried to naturally conceive unsuccessfully for three consecutive years. We tried everything from recording my menstrual cycle, ovulation kits, and even, the turkey baster method! I started questioning my own fertility and made an appointment with an OB/GYN. A laparoscopy was scheduled to discover the reason behind this three year struggle. The results came back with endometriosis-stage IV. The endometrial tissue inside my uterus was severely growing outside and plastered itself all over my fallopian tubes and ovaries. This explained the decades of excruciating chronic pain and irregular menstrual cycles as a teenager.

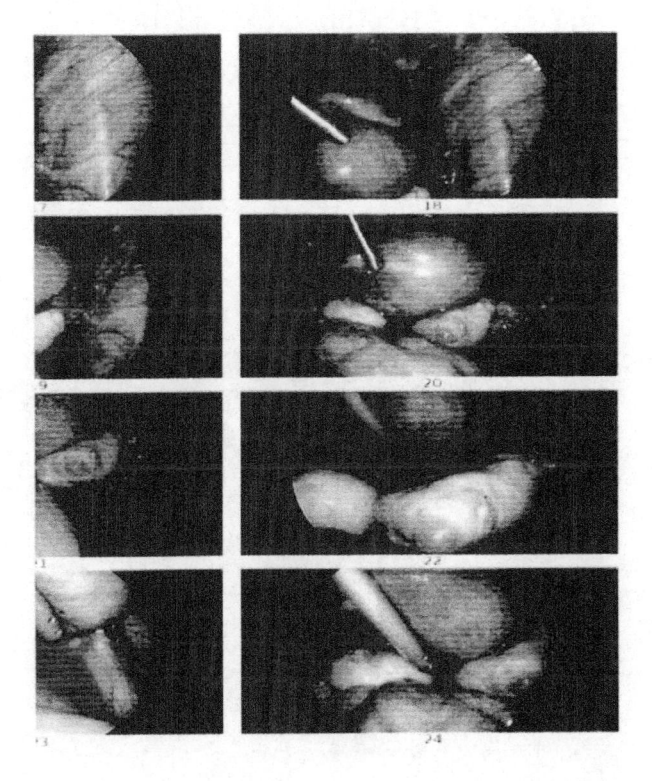

The infertility news was devastating. According to the doctor, the only way that I could conceive was via in vitro fertilization (IVF). Due to the high out of pocket expenses, physical demands, and emotional scars, we gave IVF one wholehearted chance. My Beloved husband gave me daily injections, and it became a sacred nightly ritual. There was a two-week waiting period for implantation before I could take the HCG test to see if the IVF was successful. The fertility office called with the news, "I am sorry to tell you that the test came back negative. There was no implantation." Sitting alone in my car, with an aching heart, I wailed against the steering wheel.

One question was on my mind, where do I go from here?

Feelings of anger, shame, and inadequacy consumed me. My protective dad comforted me with his words of unconditional love. "Your life still has meaning. Your life is still beautiful. Even without children, you still have a mission to fulfill." My loving mom and I tirelessly researched all about endometriosis and miraculously found a holistic and natural alternative.

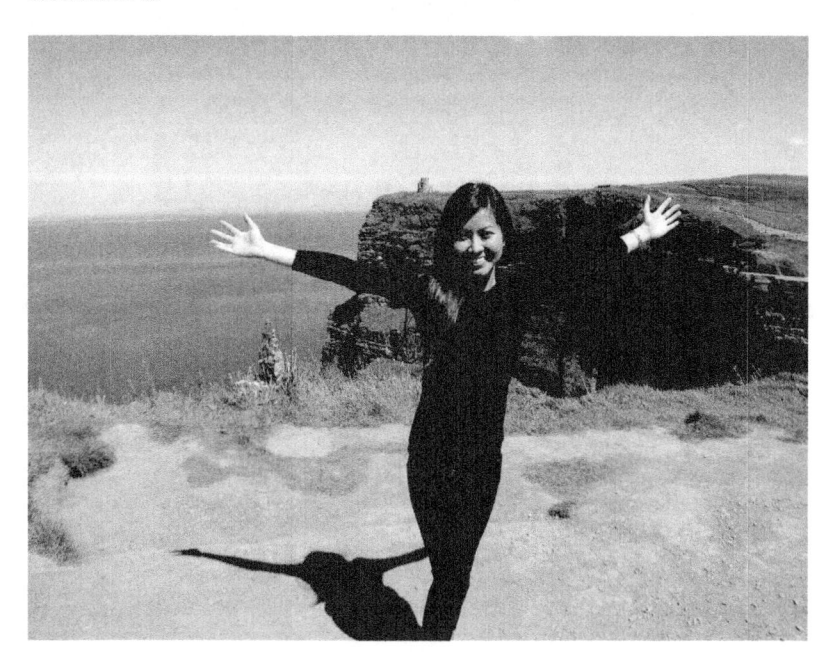

Due to the stage IV endometriosis, my body was in a highly acidic state. In order for it to reach equilibrium again, a holistic practice of only eating specific nutrient dense foods. This required mental fortitude. I committed to being my own health advocate; no one would do it for me. Steadfast, I continued with the holistic lifestyle for three months and noticed my menstrual cycle regulating itself. For the first time, my cycle came without the agonizing pain.

Tom and I accepted the fact that parenthood was not in our future. To help this grieving process, we made a resolution to enjoy life by traveling and celebrating our unconditional love for one another. That summer, Tom planned a trip for us to Ireland. It was the perfect place to ignite joy and happiness back into our lives.

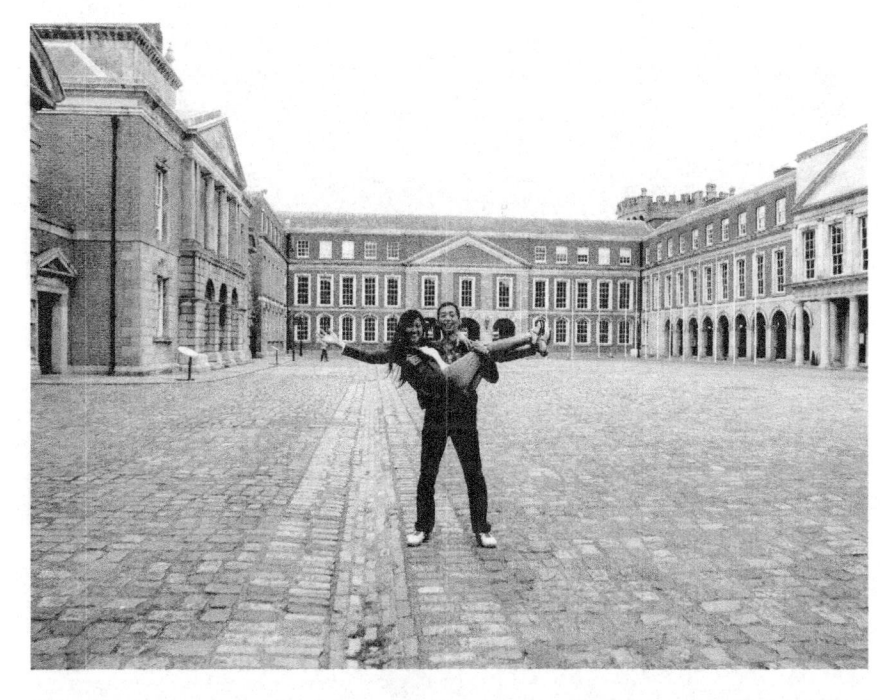

After our trip, I checked my calendar and suddenly realized that I had missed my June cycle. I dreaded that I was back to my irregular cycles and waited until July in hopes of its arrival. July came and still nothing. With a glimmer of hope, we darted to the nearest store and bought a pregnancy test. You know, the ones that are locked up behind glass doors! I could not bear to look at the results and handed it over to my husband. With hesitation, he whispered, "It's positive."

Could this be one of those false positive results? For peace of mind, we researched one of the best OB/GYN in town. He proceeded to scan my belly in search of a heartbeat. It took a while, but he finally said, "There's one heartbeat." Long pause. "And there's the second one." Overjoyed beyond belief, tears poured down our faces as Tom and I looked closer at our TWO little heartbeats.

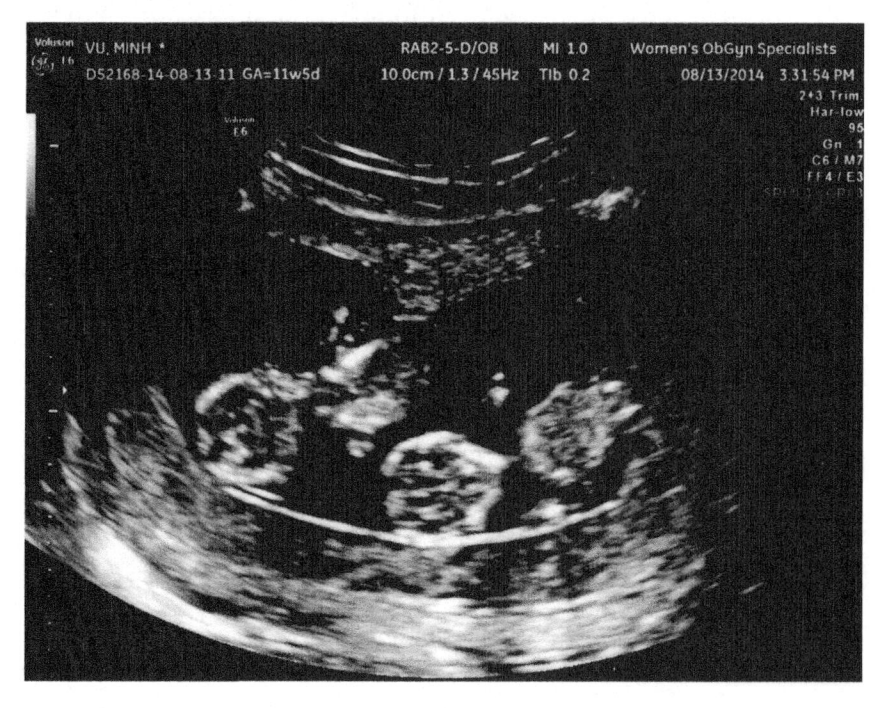

Lesson #2: God Still Performs Miracles. (Narrator: Tom Vu)

It felt like we had just won the lottery! We had already picked out the name Luke, which means Light, but were now scrambling to come up with a second memorable boy's name that began with the letter "L". Minh eventually drew inspiration from Ireland and magically came up with Liam, Protective Warrior.

One night, my wife had a dream and one of the twins was crying out, "Help me mom! I'm dying!" She vividly saw a little boy reaching out to her, while the other one was standing over his brother. Miraculously, we believe our sons were communicating with their mom at that time. I still get chills thinking about it. The very next afternoon, I rushed my wife to the emergency room due to piercing abdominal pain. Initially, Minh thought that she was having severe heartburn. It was there that we met the exemplary neonatology team made up of angels in human form, who would forever change our lives.

They informed us that my wife was experiencing one of the rare complications that we had been warned about – Twin-to-Twin Transfusion Syndrome (TTTS), Stage II. Luke was the recipient, receiving too much blood flow from the placenta; while Liam, the donor, was not receiving enough. Even in the womb, Liam lived up to his name as the protective warrior for his brother. In addition, there was excessive amniotic fluid in my wife's abdomen. Emergency fetal surgery known as Fetoscopic Laser Photocoagulation was needed immediately. They informed us that one or both of our sons may not survive, or that we may be faced with the decision of considering termination of one or both of the fetuses in order to save my wife's life.

The joy of pregnancy quickly shifted to chaos, dread, and uncertainty as I felt the world spinning out of control right before my eyes. Feeling helpless, I anxiously sat in the waiting area at the hospital with my wife's parents and frantically checked all the television monitors for any surgery status updates. Our hearts lifted when we were finally told that the surgery was successful.

When Minh was discharged, we marveled at how we had narrowly escaped adversity. After only our second day of release from the hospital, my wife noticed abnormal swelling in both of her legs while at home. We did not want to take any chances due to our past experiences and contacted her neonatologist immediately. He informed us that she was experiencing Mirror Syndrome, in which the mother and fetus both experience a buildup of fluid.

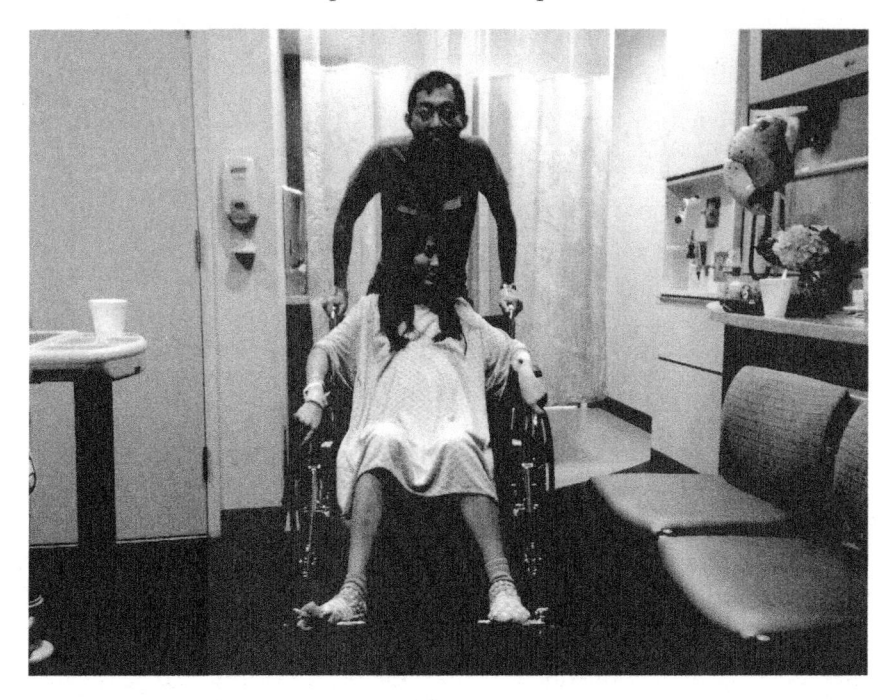

Once again, we were told that one or both sons may not survive, or that we may be faced with the decision of considering termination of one or both of the fetuses in order to save my wife's life. Miraculously, a second fetal surgery was successfully performed to transfuse blood to Liam and remove the excess fluid. After another two weeks of recovery at the hospital, my wife was discharged to go home with strict bed rest guidelines. We tried our best to make it to the 27th week gestational age that our OB/GYN was hoping for in order to give our sons the best chance for survival.

Dismally, this was not to be as we had to return to the hospital during the 26th week when my wife noticed an odd reddish-colored discharge. The hospital kept Minh there for observation. The discharge only got worse, and on our second night, Liam's heart rate quickly plummeted, while my wife was lying in a pool of her own blood.

I was asleep on the couch when a team of nurses abruptly filled the room. I felt an anxiousness and sense of urgency in the nurses' demeanor as they immediately paged her OB/GYN and directed Minh to get on her hands and knees to help raise Liam's heart rate. Our OB/GYN calmly informed us that a placental abruption had occurred, and an emergency C-section was needed immediately. On that fateful day, our amazing doctors and a team of nurses helped us welcome Light and the Protective Warrior into this world. We were absolutely madly in love with them! Luke weighed 2lbs 8oz. and little brother Liam weighed 2lbs 5oz.

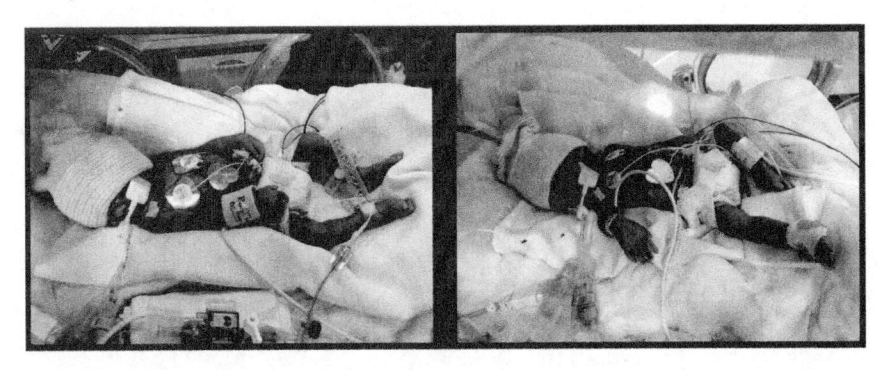

Our experience with the staff at the hospital was beyond extraordinary. We came to know them as unique and caring angels in human form, not just as healthcare workers in passing. We were profoundly moved by their compassion during our bleakest moments. Words cannot describe the immense joy that they brought into our world. They have touched our souls and will always be remembered in our hearts.

Lesson #3: Keep the faith. (Narrator: Minh Vu)

Where I was afraid of:

> ...being broken, I was simply in need of God's love, self-love, and inner-healing.
> ...being rejected, I learned to never reject myself.

…being abandoned, I learned to never abandon myself.

…other's opinions, I learned that my own carried more weight.

…painful endings, I learned that they were actually new beginnings.

…being seen as small and insignificant, I discovered my potent power.

…being perceived as less than, I realized I was more than enough.

…being perceived as ugly, I learned to fully embrace my own beauty.

…feeling low, I learned that it was the birth of divine brilliance.

…change, I realized that it was an inevitable part of life.

…being alone, I learned to savor and relish my own company.

…life itself, I rediscovered who I truly am.

…hopelessness, I experienced God's supernatural miracles that surpassed all understanding.

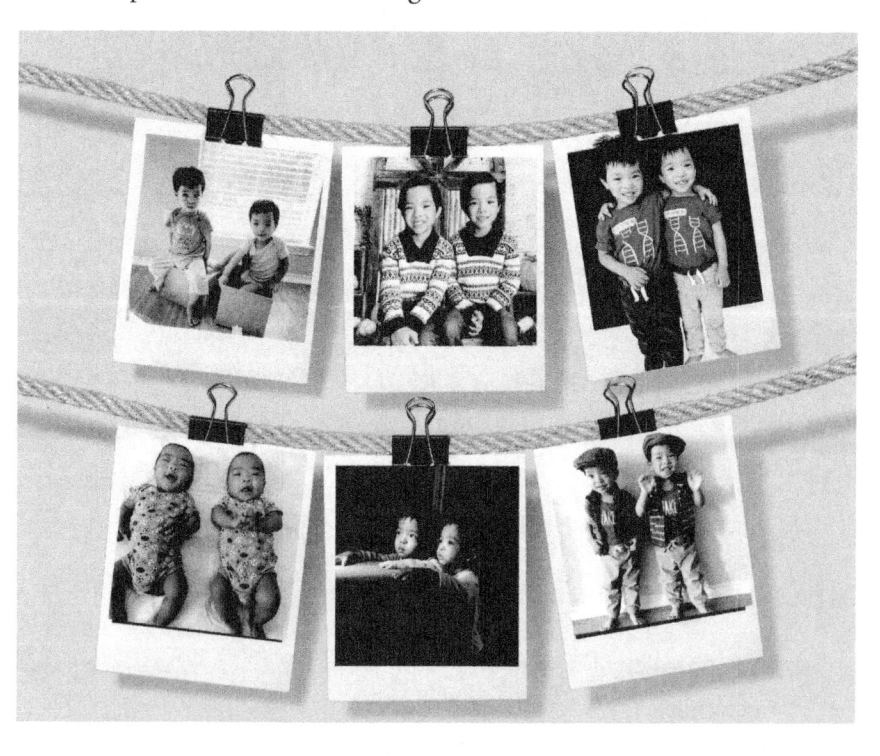

My Beloved Endo-Sisters and Fertility-Sisters, keep the faith. If I can conquer stage 4 endometriosis, infertility, a failed IVF, and so much more to bring my miracle babies into this world, so can you! Take faith-filled action steps toward your wildest dreams. Let me empower you in your holistic freedom journey, I personally invite you to connect with me at endotransformation.com or minh@endotransformation.com

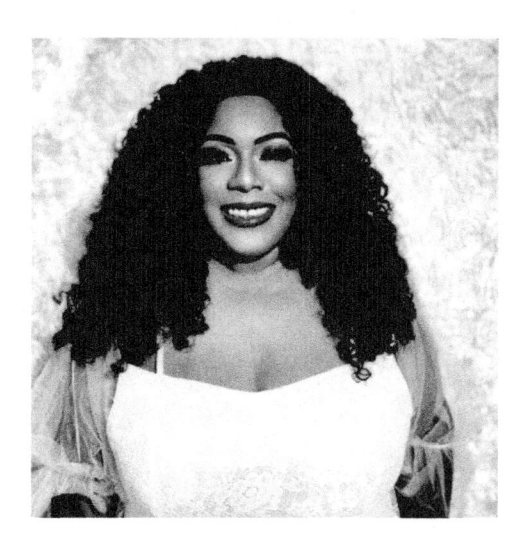

Charlotte Howard Collins

Heart Centered Women Publishing
Female Business Growth Expert

www.linkedin.com/in/charlottehoward
www.instagram.com/coachwithcharlotte
www.facebook.com/charlottehoward
www.charlottehowardcollins.com
www.heartcenteredwomenpublishing.com

Award Winning Female Business Growth Expert, Best Selling Author, Publisher, Producer, BookToker, Speaker, and Self-Made Entrepreneur, Charlotte Howard Collins works with small businesswomen to multi-millionaire and billionaire female entrepreneurs developing business growth systems, sales processes, competition-crushing marketing, compelling offers, and client experiences.

She is the CEO of Wealthy Women Enterprises, Wealthy Women Inner Circle, Wealthy Women Entrepreneurs Network, Hair Artist Association, and Heart Centered Women Publishing. She helps her clients generate immediate increases in revenue and profits… without spending an additional cent on marketing or advertising! Charlotte and her clients have been featured in thousands of magazines and media outlets. She is a loving wife and mom to four beautiful children! In her spare time, she loves hairstyling, exercising, relaxing on the beach, traveling, reading, and writing."

LIVE A FULLY CHARGED LIFE TODAY

By Charlotte Howard Collins

"Leave nothing for tomorrow which can be done today."
—Abraham Lincoln

This must be a quote you have heard a hundred times before. There is, of course, a kind of simplicity in how these nine words convey a simple message – don't put things off for later.

Are you one of those people who always put off things for later? Well, you are not alone. This is a problem that almost everyone goes through at least once in their life.

Among the things that make individuals happy is the company of loved ones and friends. I am glad I had my mom and second dad in my life for a long time, even when some of my family and friends turned their backs on me. The dynamic backup my mom, dad, and daughter gave me was priceless.

You probably don't enjoy being smothered by your family, but getting together for an occasional cookout increases your happiness. Having individuals around you that you love, trust, cherish, and care for makes you feel that you're not alone.

I lost my biological father in a terrible car accident at eight years old. His funeral was on my birthday. Years ago, when we had our cookouts, it felt different because my biological father's brother had passed away. It felt like my birth father dying all over again. He used to take us to Disney world every year when we were younger, and when we got older he joined us for cookouts every year. He never put it off. He traveled from New Jersey to see us and always had the latest and greatest movies and stories to share.

You may feel a little hesitant when opening your life up to others. You may not want to open yourself up because you are uncomfortable with new people or have mistrusted people in the past, but you need to find ways to overcome the issues and open your heart to others.

You will find that sustaining and maintaining friendships and relationships can be challenging, but sometimes you must take chances. You never know what a relationship or friendship might bring you in the future, but one thing is for sure, you need to learn how to get over the past and live for the future.

Now look toward the ground and notice if any ropes are holding you down, stopping you from being free to fly. To go on in your life, it is necessary to cut those ropes—to overcome not your fears of failure, but your fears of success.

When it comes to your inner energy, you will find that you have all the strength to get up and achieve or seek out whatever makes you happy. It would be best if you tried to seek out a happy, healthy, and fulfilling life. When your time is up, you will want to be able to say that you've done it all. However, many people fear the end because of all there is that they want to seek.

Why not leave a legacy for your family?

What is it that you wish to seek out? It would be best if you defined what you want so that you can dig up all the energy inside to help you achieve your goals. You should also try to realize what type of energy you have and how to tap the energy out of you when you seek a plan.

First, would you say that you are normally an optimistic or pessimistic person regarding the overall attitude of your life? If you find yourself positive, you should consider yourself fortunate not to let others drag you down. If you are negative, you need to find ways to turn your negative into a positive.

One way to convert your energy is to seek a massage therapist. That's right, a massage therapist, especially one that specializes in Reiki massage. This massage allows all your negative energy out and fills you with hope, peace, and love. Not to mention it will help you with your goals in life.

You will find that when your energy has been cleansed, you will be able to carry on with your life with all intentions of reaching for the stars. When you have positive energy, you will find the strength to do anything; now, all you have to do is use it.

How can you tap into your energy to help you deal with some of your goals and the obstacles you need to pass? Well, the only way to use it is to realize that you have the power to do whatever your heart desires and that you allow yourself to reach your goals.

To get the energy to meet a life-changing goal, you need to know that you can do it and have to have passion. It is the passion that will make your goals obtainable. You need to want it so bad that you have to do it. If you want something that badly, nothing will get in your way. All you have to do is know what you want out of life. If you can define what you want, you will be able to achieve all that you have set in mind.

Once you define your goals and who you are, the picture will be much clearer. You will notice that your dreams will seem to become closer, and you will be able to work your way up to more goals. When you hit a rough spot, you have two options; either push forward or quit.

Do you want to quit, or do you want to see it through? If you have passion, your decision would be to keep going. You will find a way to meet your goals and have everything you ever dreamed of come true. However, it is hard, and you must put in the effort. If it is something that you genuinely want, then you will find a way to achieve it.

It's all about living your best life, having been through it all.

To live your best life, you need to take care of your mind, body, and soul. When all three are in alignment, you'll find personal success comes more easily. It takes courage to live your best life—the courage to be authentic to yourself. This can be scary, but it's also incredibly freeing. You'll find the motivation and inspiration you need to pursue your dreams when you're living your best life. Everything will fall into place when you're living in alignment with your deepest values and passions. So don't be afraid to go after what you want in life—go after your dreams with everything you've got. You deserve to live your best life, mind, body, and soul.

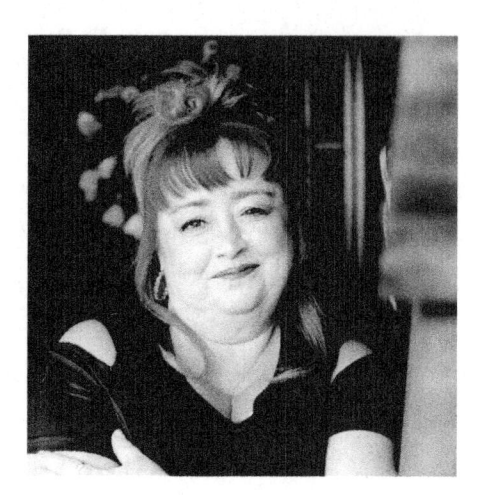

A. Michelle Bell

Co-Founder of Health Business Boss Institute

https://www.linkedin.com/company/virtual-work-wife
https://www.instagram.com/virtualworkwife/
https://www.facebook.com/virtualworkwife
https://healthbossinstitute.com
https://www.virtualworkwife.com

Michelle is CEO of Virtual Work Wife and Co-Founder of Health Business Boss Institute.

The Institute provides business coaching, automation training, and consulting support to female entrepreneurs, fitness professionals, health, and lifestyle coaches who want to create successful streams of income that allow them to profit from their passion and pursue a life guided by the communities they engage with.

Their signature system is a 13-week program designed to help you get clear on what makes YOU unique, how to productize and monetize your skillset, and how to build a strong foundation through automation to share your message with the world.

Michelle has an intuitive sense of what YOUR business needs in order to provide authentic and genuine experiences that will turn YOUR clients into superfans.

When she's not teaching, speaking or on the road for dance competitions, Michelle enjoys time spent at home with her family in Jamul, California.

FROM TOTAL HEALTH TRANSFORMATION TO FINANCIAL FREEDOM

By A. Michelle Bell

Most people dive into health or wellness coaching do so because they experienced a life-changing health crisis, personally or through a loved one. The event inspired taking action and ignited a passion for helping others, which is amazing. I mean, we all love an inspirational hero's story, right?!?

Some might quit a full-time job to pursue life as a Coach or retire and find purpose in a second career as a solopreneur, changing the face of healthcare one client at a time. But all too quickly they realize there's a limit to how many people they can help and still work on their business and sustain a livable income.

That's what I want to talk about today. How you can save time and make more money as a health and wellness advocate.

Kind of a cool subject, right?

You're probably wondering who I am and why you should listen to me, so let's take a beat and I'll tell you a little about myself.

My name is Michelle and I'm a marketing strategist, coach, speaker, and author. I've owned multiple six-figure businesses and consulted for Fortune 100 companies. But most of all I'm a mom.

My health coach told me to stop spending so much time at work. I was sacrificing balance and rest trying to juggle career and family.

In 2005 I quit corporate life to follow my passion: helping people build their businesses and work on their own terms.

Work is like… you know… *work*. And who wants to spend 12+ hours a day doing that?!

I prioritized creating balance. Truthfully, it was easy because work should never come before family. Or, for the single ladies, those things you need to feel fulfilled.

Putting family first and business second is the best decision of my life. I'm present every day for my kids.

If you've never said, "Do you want mommy to get a real job? Because I will," can you even call yourself a mompreneur? 😊

Where were we? Right, we want to reduce errors, create wow-worthy client experiences, save time and make more money.

It's all possible when you fix your fulfillment!

You might be thinking: But Michelle, I don't sell "widgets" this doesn't apply to me… but it does! Delivering client onboarding is just as important, if not more so, than delivering a physical product. And just as likely to result in bad reviews!!

Fulfillment isn't just shipping products. Fulfillment is how clients meet with you, interact with your content, and how _they deliver items to you_.

You may think of this as customer service. But when you shift your thinking into fulfilling services, you begin to see how much time and money you can save by automating workflow.

Happy customers become brand ambassadors. Your Cheerleaders. Your SALESFORCE.

When you fix your fulfillment and deliver WOW, you positively impact your bottom line and set yourself up to gain repeat buyers.

Happy, satisfied customers are more likely to repurchase _from you_ over a brand or person they don't know.

When it comes to health and wellness, average buyers are way more cautious. Scripts and gimmicks don't fool them. They are cultivated through sharing similar experiences, they build trust by empathizing with authentic stories.

Why do so few businesses keep the customers that they already have? Most of the time it's because *they don't know how to retain the customer*.

They don't know how to improve the client experience in order to make that person repurchase. They don't have processes in place to drive the client to the next step.

Meaning, as soon as someone does what you asked – attend sessions, complete worksheets, etc. - what is the next action they should take, and how do they get there?

Most people hire a coach or consultant because they want to be led. They want to be educated. **They want you to grab them by hand and drag them to their success.**

They want you to fix all their problems. The same is true for sales.

They want you to tell them what to buy next, and if you don't have an offer in place, they won't take action. Or worse, they go to a competitor.

So what's keeping you from working less and having more profit in your coaching business?

Here are some common problems …

- inconsistent delivery because you're manually tracking sessions sold or freebies promised.
- hit-and-miss capture of agreements or documents because you're creating them as you go.
- You'd love to be better at welcoming new buyers or sharing content, but you don't know how.

The solution …. Automation

Remember, fulfillment is the process of delivering what you've already sold. This can be:

- Using a dispensary or warehouse
- Using a membership site to provide content
- Using a CRM to automate onboarding

Automation streamlines your processes so everyone gets the right content at the right time for the right purpose.

Your clients will feel supported and have WOW moments with less overall work on your part, which keeps your costs low. When the time is right to turn your clients into repeat buyers you will know who is hot and ready to see your offers.

Let's face it, no one likes making sales calls. Imagine if your clients saw the right offer at the right time and simply clicked "add to cart". #amazeballs

Automation is like having a virtual assistant. When done right, it saves you time, creates growth, and saves money in lead generation and retention costs. AND, once set up, it runs completely on autopilot.

It Helps Your Customers, Too!

They receive targeted content that supports their journey toward a goal. Not just purchase goals, but personal growth goals, too. It helps them become invested in your ecosystem, access more content, build trust in your business, and deliver value so they feel seen and supported. This is how clients become superfans … aka… referral partners!

So How Do You Make It Happen?

Well, it starts with a plan! What you need is a good map. No, not like the one in grandpa's glove box. A map of your ideal customer experience from the moment they find you to their fifth, sixth, or tenth purchase.

BONUS!

I have this nifty handout for you. It's full of the most common pitstops along the map of coaching.

https://virtualworkwife.com/fulfillment

Next, You Need a Good CRM (Contact Relationship Management System)

My favorite is Keap, but there are plenty of options. When it comes to creating your map you want something without limitations.

Set up your onboarding workflow with actions and goals for you AND your client. For example, when a purchase is made …

- Send an email explaining what will happen next.
- Track customer progress and look for outliers, people who DIDN'T do what's expected.
- Move completed buyers to your next offer and get testimonials!

Getting your client to sign a program agreement is a great place to start. No need for expensive tools, a simple "by signing this agreement…" statement on an ordinary web form can do the trick.

BONUS!

Need a program agreement? No problem! I got you boo:

https://virtualworkwife.com/agreement-template

Remember, this is a sample. I highly recommend having your attorney look it over. 😊

By automating onboarding, your CRM acts as a babysitter. It monitors client progress for you. **IF** they get stuck, the CRM alerts you to step in and get them unstuck.

Another great automation is delivering and collecting forms. As a coach, you may need …

- Lifestyle or medical history
- Supplement or dietary logs

Letting the CRM automatically send the proper form at the right time and then hold the person until it's completed allows you to stay focused and work with those who are ready for the next step.

> **Pro Tip**: Most CRMs have form-building functionalities and can integrate with tools like Survey Monkey or Jotform.

It is essential to know how many people you have on your map and their progress. It lets you know when you have enough clients and when it's time to add more.

It tells you when to offer upsells. What would it mean to your bottom line if you could automatically offer every client who finishes your program an upsell to monthly maintenance?

What could an extra $100 per month per person mean for your financial health?

Who's been to a fast-food joint where they turned that iPad-style register around to ask you for a tip? Can you still feel all eyes on you from that experience… #sothedrama

Do you feel the same about asking clients for money? Automating the "ask" makes it less cringy. They don't have you watching them decide and you don't have to pretend to be chill while internally screaming; just buy it already!

Now… the big question. Are you going to implement automation in your business?

Would it be easier if this was mapped out and done for you?
(I bet it would!)

> **BONUS:** My FREE Automation Audit helps you take the first step toward automating your business. www.virtualworkwife.com/work-with-us

SCAN ME
Bonus #3 - FREE Consultation

We'll go through exactly what you're already doing
- on whatever platform you're already using - and I'll show you at least three places to improve. This could be how to…

- automatically find your hottest leads for personalized follow-up
- shorten onboarding time with new clients
- ensure your list is full of only engaged, excited prospects
- follow up after your leads take action
- re-engage leads who "abandon cart"

Or one of the hundreds of ways I know to capture more sales with automation.

One conversation can change your life.

JOIN THE MOVEMENT!
#BAUW

Becoming An Unstoppable Woman With She Rises Studios

She Rises Studios was founded by Hanna Olivas and Adriana Luna Carlos, the mother-daughter duo, in mid-2020 as they saw a need to help empower women around the world. They are the podcast hosts of the *She Rises Studios Podcast* as well as Amazon best-selling authors and motivational speakers who travel the world. Hanna and Adriana are the movement creators of #BAUW - Becoming An Unstoppable Woman: The movement has been created to universally impact women of all ages, at whatever stage of life, to overcome insecurities, and adversities, and develop an unstoppable mindset. She Rises Studios educates, celebrates, and empowers women globally.

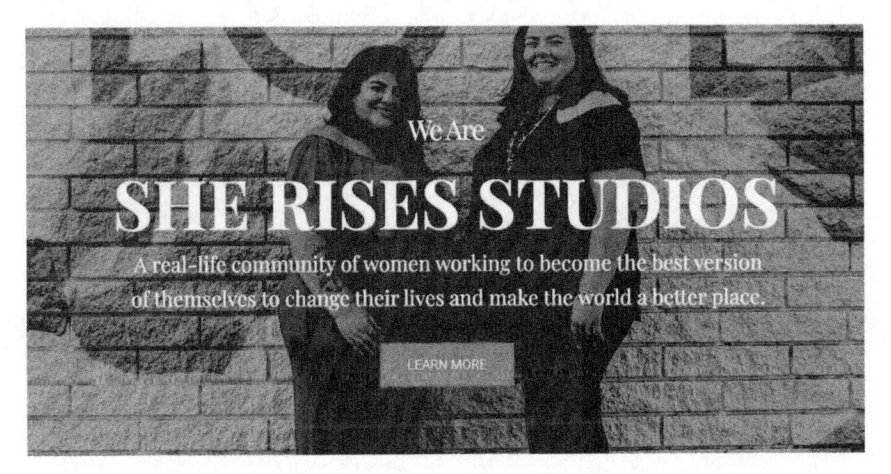

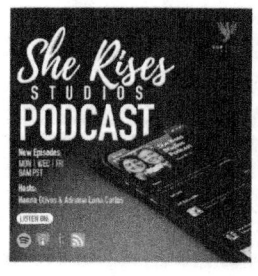

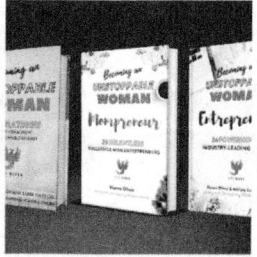

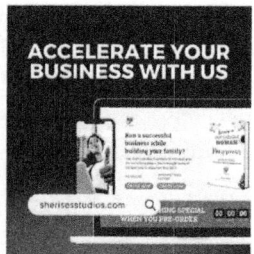

Looking to Join Us in our Next Anthology or Publish YOUR Own?

She Rises Studios Publishing offers full-service publishing, marketing, book tour, and campaign services. For more information, contact info@sherisesstudios.com

We are always looking for women who want to share their stories and expertise and feature their businesses on our podcasts, in our books, and in our magazines.

SEE WHAT WE DO

OUR PODCAST　　**OUR BOOKS**　　**OUR SERVICES**

Be featured in the Becoming An Unstoppable Woman magazine, published in 13 countries and sold in all major retailers. Get the visibility you need to LEVEL UP in your business!

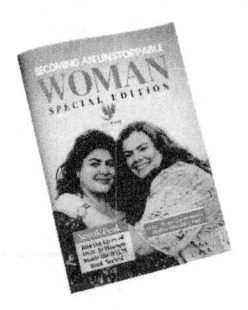

Visit www.SheRisesStudios.com to see how YOU can join the #BAUW movement and help your community to achieve the UNSTOPPABLE mindset.

Have you checked out the *She Rises Studios Podcast?*

Find us on all MAJOR platforms: Spotify, IHeartRadio, Apple Podcasts, Google Podcasts, etc.

Looking to become a sponsor or build a partnership?

Email us at info@sherisesstudios.com

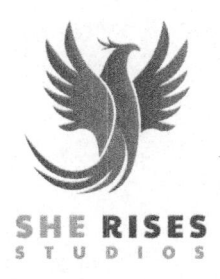

SHE RISES
STUDIOS

Printed by Amazon Italia Logistica S.r.l.
Torrazza Piemonte (TO), Italy